Language of the Feet

written by

Chris Stormer
SRN, SCM, HV, RT

Illustrated by

Michele Shayne Davey

Hodder Education

AN HACHETTE UK COMPANY

Orders: Please contact Bookpoint Ltd, 130 Milton Park, Abingdon, Oxon OX14 4SB.
Telephone: (44) 01235 827720, Fax: (44) 01235 400454.
Lines are open from 9.00 to 5.00, Monday to Saturday, with a 24-hour message
answering service. You can also order through our website
www.hoddereducation.co.uk.

British Library Cataloguing in Publication Data
A catalogue record for this title is available from the British Library.

ISBN-13: 978 0 340 93959 8

First published   2007
Impression number   10 9 8 7 6 5
Year   2012 2011

Typeset by Transet Ltd., Coventry, England.
Printed in Great Britain for Hodder Education, an Hachette Livre UK Company,
338 Euston Road, London NW1 3BH by CPI Cox & Wyman Ltd, Reading,
Berkshire, RG1 8EX.

Hachette Livre UK's policy is to use papers that are natural, renewable and recyclable
products and made from wood grown in sustainable forests. The logging and
manufacturing processes are expected to conform to the environmental regulations of
the country of origin.

Contents

Dedication

For all the tremendous souls in my life, particularly John, Andrew
and David.

Introduction

There is far more to the feet than first meets the eye!

The English language abounds with numerous references to feet, such as 'standing on one's own two feet', 'getting a foot in the door', 'footing the bill' and so on, yet, on the whole, scant attention is paid to them; that is, until they hurt. When this happens, it is difficult to think straight, let alone get on with anything important. In fact, the discomfort can be so unbearable that everything can come to a complete standstill. It's the body's way of saying that something is drastically wrong. Even though the body constantly conveys messages, it is not always clear what it is trying to 'say', which is where the feet step in. By highlighting the more pertinent aspects of ongoing mind chatter, feet are quick to reveal any threat to personal well-being; whilst, at the same time, they happily deal with adversities that could get in the way. Even though feet are relatively small compared to the rest of the body, they have phenomenal strength and are in an excellent position to carry mind, body and soul from place to place. As they do so, they frequently take on the weight of the mind, as well as hefty emotional issues that trouble the soul.

Knowing the basic language that feet speak helps to create a deeper awareness of what's going on at ground level, providing much-needed guidance into knowing which steps to take to become even better at being oneself. This assistance is particularly useful when constantly being tripped up by the same old problems that just don't seem to go away. Yet the greatest problem is that of not knowing what it is that was so upsetting in the first place, since most issues tend to stem from long-forgotten memories, with their pitiful remnants niggling at the back of the mind. Until they are mentally dealt with, the uneasiness can make one so sick that it ultimately develops into some dreaded unease or 'dis-ease'. The medical profession are well aware of how feet mirror overall health, frequently using them to detect the early signs of certain illnesses such as diabetes and arthritis, as well as many neurological and circulatory conditions. This book shares this knowledge in simple, everyday language and spells out the many fascinating and insightful ways in which feet constantly change their characteristics to get their

✱ 9

message across. Some changes are barely noticeable, whilst others can be painfully obvious, especially when the impact of daily events leave their mark on one's personality and feet. Those experiences that stand out the most and make the greatest impression on the soul generally show up on the soles, especially when rigid belief systems get in the way.

A great deal can be attained from feet, such as why toenails are painted, why toe rings are worn and why alluring ankle chains hang around this part of the body, as well as reasons for some of the discreet, or not-so-discreet, tattoos. It may be a little more difficult to understand why some women choose to mutilate their feet by having their third toes amputated so that they can force their feet into fashionably pointed shoes in the vain hope of gaining acceptance in an often callous society. Yet, there are also those who prefer to be footloose and fancy-free and invariably go around barefoot. The feet are really grateful for these opportunities 'to breathe', particularly if they spend most of the time feeling gagged in the constraining confines of socks or stockings and then heartlessly being shoved into the cramped confines of shoes that have exceptionally high temperatures and often equally high odours. It's hardly surprising that feet are prone to complain from time to time.

There is also an extensive metaphysical side to feet, long known by many indigenous cultures, as well as some Eastern health practitioners, who frequently use the important messages conveyed by the feet to determine the best possible approach for ongoing health. They do this by looking at the sizes and shapes of the toes, to determine the capacity to think; they study areas with hard skin, to decide which parts are being put to the test; they look at the curvature of arches, to gain insight into the amount of inner strength and personal resourcefulness, and so on. Feet continually grow or shrink even during adulthood, depending on whether there is a willingness to cover new ground or a tendency to shirk and pull back. Feet also have much to say about how the quality of life impacts on the mental, physical, emotional and spiritual balance of the individual. The 'Language of the Feet' provides a remarkable glimpse into the intricate workings of the elusive subconscious mind, since it is this that is responsible for changing the characteristics of the feet, such as their shape to highlight the shape of things to come, as well as their size to reveal the impression made every time the foot is put down. This book provides the ideal opportunity to finally let go of dreadful memories that keep getting in the way, making it so much easier to move on, although in the process an array of conflicting emotions, ranging from utter disbelief and complete denial to absolute wonderment and total conviction, may be evoked. The temptation to dismiss certain parts of the book as complete 'nonsense' is a natural reaction when there is a deep-seated fear of facing innermost demons, which are dreadful memories that rear their ugly heads from time to time. Read about the feet with an open, non-judgmental mind and see how the meaningful suggestions offered can improve the quality of life; after all, it's so much easier to stride ahead when you're healthy. Fortunately reading the feet is really simple!

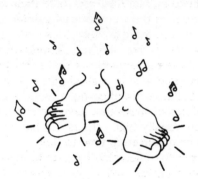

FEET BRING BALANCE BACK INTO LIFE

01 Watch the feet!

A CLOSER LOOK AT FEET

Feet are integral to overall well-being.

Feet are generally considered to be useful in moving the body from one experience to the next, as well as an extremely helpful way of getting a feel for the progress being made in life. Yet feet are also the roots and foundation upon which everybody gets to know themselves better. As messengers of the body, they willingly carry the impressions of all that goes on at soul level by simply changing their appearance. Just by glancing at them, it's amazing how easy it is to get a gist of what they are trying to portray. In time, it becomes increasingly clear how they provide endless clues as to what is going on on the inside, so that the most appropriate steps can be taken on the outside. This is why those in the healing profession frequently use feet to determine the most suitable remedy, as well as the best ways in which to conserve good health. Amongst the many aspects that they are interested in is the condition of the skin, which helps determine exactly what it is that gets under the skin for the best solution to be found. Furthermore the skin colouring (page 93) constantly fluctuates, highlighting and mirroring the ever-changing emotions that, if too intense for too long, can become highly toxic and seriously interfere with one's health. The good news is that just by acknowledging that these noxious notions exist is sufficient for things to start settling down and, in the long run, prevent disease. Then again, even though footwear (page 201) is frequently blamed for foot disorders, it is becoming increasingly evident that the body uses external measures, such as these, to attract attention to some deep constraints and constrictions that desperately need addressing. There is all this and so much more to look for when ascertaining exactly what is a-foot!

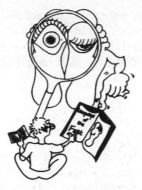

THERE IS FAR MORE THAN FIRST MEETS THE EYE!

REFLECTED ONTO THE FEET

The first step in reading feet is to get to know how the content or discontent of the mind affects the various parts of the body and the way in which these are reflected onto the feet. It is then so much easier to know what is going on, especially when there is a buildup of discontent playing havoc with the inside of the body. Trouble really starts with the pretence that everything is okay, yet, deep down, knowing that it isn't since the ever-elusive subconscious mind is inclined to hang on to a whole host of out-dated beliefs, frightful memories, unresolved hurts, unanswered questions, deep resentment, festering anger and so on. In time these can become really toxic to the mind and make the body sick.

Fortunately, feet draw attention to troublesome areas long before they become an issue and cause problems in the body. In so doing they reveal the root of the matter, not to blame but recognize the horrific memories or constraining beliefs that can get in the way of health and well-being. Blaming outside one's self for misfortune and illness really doesn't help, since it puts the power and ability to do something beneficial beyond reach, which can make it very difficult to do anything worthwhile to improve the situation. However, a lot of 'good' can and does come from something 'bad', especially when it no longer gets on the nerves. Once the issue is resolved in the mind, the irritant need never disturb or cause any further discomfort in the body. It's by sorting out the remnants of the past that the individual feels increasingly better about themselves and others, which then makes it possible for them to move from victim mood to good health. Once it is acknowledged that nobody and nothing is a threat, unless allowed to be, then it becomes increasingly effortless to enjoy the gift of the now and step confidently into the future.

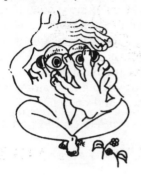

IT'S LAME TO BLAME!

How to get started

To understand feet start by looking at your own feet and invite others to do the same. Be aware of your thoughts as soon as you catch sight of them and determine what you particularly like or dislike about them. Then describe any parts that may be too painful to look at or any specific changes that would make them look better. In this way, it's possible to work out what's going on at ground level and whether you and others are getting ahead in the way that you should. It also brings to the fore problematic areas as well as uncomfortable aspects. Much can be discovered by constantly questioning and by turning the answers into the next question. For instance, if feet are considered to be 'ugly', determine what 'ugly' means to the person concerned and what it is that makes them appear 'ugly'. Should 'ugly' mean 'horrible, unpleasant or not very nice' and the 'ugly' part of the feet be a 'crooked third toe' on the 'right foot', then find out what connotations are linked to 'crooked'. If 'crooked' implies 'not being straight', then question whether anybody was 'not straight' about what was being done or not done in the 'past', since the 'right third toe' reflects thoughts about previous incidences. Alternatively, a crooked third toe could imply a situation that wasn't as straightforward as expected, which still throws one off track. There are numerous other possible explanations each with their own interpretation based on personal memories and beliefs. So it is, that a part of the foot that is particularly disliked invariably highlights hateful memories, usually with hefty emotional tags, whilst the more lovable aspects of feet reveal innermost qualities that the individual feels good about. Constant questioning identifies those things that still niggle at the back of the mind and are difficult to put a finger on. Throughout the journey through life, thoughts and feelings do change, and as they do so, so too do the characteristics of the feet, along with one's acceptance or rejection of them and oneself.

Here are a few examples of what feet can be portraying.

- Feet are tucked out of sight:
  - due to embarrassment
  - to avoid criticism
  - from being very shy
  - because of needing time out
  - to keep oneself to oneself.

- Stretching the feet out in front of oneself, when sitting, reveals:
  - how good one feels about oneself
  - one has no qualms about what others think or say
  - the need to put out feelers, make an impression or get out there.

Anything that disturbs the status quo immediately shows up on the feet long before disturbing the body, since feet are the sounding boards of the body. As such they continually draw attention to possible threats, through aches, pains, deformities and so on, in the hope that they can be nipped in the bud and momentum re-established. So, to know what the reflexes on the feet are trying to 'say', keep in mind that there are endless possibilities, only a few of which can be mentioned in this book. Rather, trust your instincts and go with your gut feel, whilst giving your imagination free reign. Your intuition, which is often referred to as your inner tutor, will show you the way. The more you trust it the stronger it becomes, helping you to determine what is really going on at a much deeper level. This makes it so much easier to come up with a solution since these reside within the body. Only the individual concerned really knows how best to improve their situation; nobody else can do it for them!

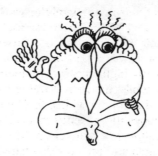

THOUGHTS ABOUT FEET.

THE IMPACT OF DEMANDING SITUATIONS

Thankfully, nobody leads the perfect life! Contrary to popular belief, it would be so boring! Yet, ironically, everybody does, in their own peculiar way, lead the 'perfect' life – 'perfect' for them that is! Each individual subconsciously creates their own reality, at soul level, helping them to understand that challenges are opportunities to become better at being oneself and that life is an exciting adventure of self-discovery. The stresses and strains are a chance to rediscover innermost capabilities and resourcefulness and it is often the most demanding situation that becomes the most exhilarating experience, bringing to the fore untried and untested talents, thereby strengthening the inner core. When it comes to reacting to distressing circumstances there are choices of what to do or not do. The option to succumb and be overwhelmed can eventually lead to constant tiredness and sickness, whereas the choice to get on top of a frightful situation is generally far more rewarding and worthwhile! Either way there are always consequences, since whatever is put into life is exactly what comes out of it. Even though frustrating and infuriating situations can and do constantly get in the way, they are simply testing points, that used advantageously, can be extremely beneficial. Feet are in the ideal position to detect what is going on underfoot and show that whatever happens, the situation is perfect for personal growth and ongoing development!

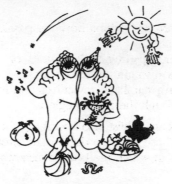

ENJOYING THE PRESENT.

NOTE

The language of the feet is useful in making the best decisions and bringing about beneficial changes in attitude that can ultimately create the 'perfect' life.

UNDERSTANDING FEET

Feet may be relatively small in relation to the rest of the body but they are incredibly versatile and resilient. Being ideally designed to carry the whole body, they easily adapt to ongoing needs and provide ongoing insight and understanding. The word 'under-stand' is intriguing since feet are 'under' the body and are used to 'stand' on, which is why they are so aware of all that goes on above them whilst willingly taking on weighty thoughts and hefty emotions to show what's afoot. No matter how much is dumped on them feet do everything in their power to keep the body upright and mobile. By staying firmly on the ground, the head can be held up high and the body can then benefit from the extremes that come its way, which show up on the feet as follows:

- The toes and toe necks reflect the head and neck revealing the impact of thoughts, that are ethereal by nature.
- The balls of the feet show how emotions, kept close to the chest, fill the surrounding air with each breath.

- The upper halves of the insteps exhibit how the passion of doing things stems from the 'belly'.
- The lower halves of the insteps imitate the fluidity of communications that flow through the lower gut.
- The heels reveal how earth stabilizes, revitalizes and motivates mind, body and spirit through the pelvic region.

Feet ground all these elements, whilst also absorbing the necessary resources from the earth. These are then distributed throughout to supplement the other ways in which the body constantly recharges itself.

- The body refreshes itself through air breathed in and out through the lungs.
- It re-energizes itself from the warmth of the sun, via the hairs on the body.
- It uses food, taken in via the digestive tract, to invigorate the whole being.

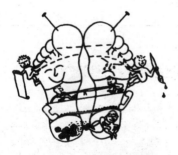

INSIGHT GAINED FROM THE MEANINGS OF THE FEET.

STEPS TO READING THE FEET

Reading feet can be an absolute eye-opener, which is why, when combined with Reflexology (an ancient art of massaging feet) the outcome can be phenomenal. Merging the two intensifies the effect of the therapeutic movements and powerfully augments healing. Yet it is inevitable that throughout life, things do go 'wrong', which provides the chance to reassess dreadful memories and inhibiting beliefs that keep getting in the way. These generally show up on the feet before affecting the body. Even though the skin on the soles does tend to be thicker, these parts are highly sensitive due to the high density of nerves. By drawing energy from the ground, they keep mind, body and soul in tip-top condition, which is why tension in the body can cause havoc. It causes the muscles in the feet to tighten, which immediately restricts the flow of life force energy throughout the feet, as well as the whole body. With cells becoming progressively deprived, the body and feet become increasingly vulnerable and susceptible to disorders and disease. Yet, once the mind lets go of fear, the body and feet can relax and, once again, powerfully draw upon external energies. The relief of letting go of so many unnecessary burdens is enormous; body, mind and spirit can completely relax and get on with what they do best, which is to keep themselves fit, healthy and happy. It is through the appreciation of life that the present becomes so much more manageable and healing can really begin.

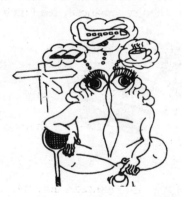

No idea which way to turn?

Taking a step at a time

Reading feet is surprisingly simple because, on some level, everybody knows how to do it and just needs reminding. It can, however, be highly emotive since baring the soles is symbolic of baring the soul, which is why it is necessary to be sensitive and really careful in the choice of words used. Rather than being judgemental, condemning or critical, try to keep an open mind and be intuitively guided. Start by seating the individual comfortably in front of you with their bare soles at eye level, ensuring that there is sufficient light, preferably natural, directly on them. Warn the individual that some deep-seated emotions may be evoked during the reading but that this is good and reassure them that they are in safe hands.

When first looking at the feet, make a mental note of your initial reaction and be conscious of feelings that are stirred since these give clues as to the individual's true spirit and provide useful insight into what is going on at a much deeper level. Then ask them to tense their feet by squeezing them tightly, which tends to accentuate distressed areas, that tend to turn bright red or a creamy whitish yellow. These patches reveal deeply-suppressed emotions that are likely to erupt when under pressure or when the squeeze is on. Next invite the individual to stretch their toes and open their feet as wide as possible to determine which emotions are most likely to surface when overly stretched. Then systematically read their feet, keeping the following in mind:

- Check whether both feet look similar, if not, note how they differ (page 171), since this reveals differences between their past and current circumstances.
- The relationship of the pair of feet (page 168) is a gauge to the amount of give and take in their lives.
- The angle of the feet (page 98) establishes the perimeters within which the individual functions.
- The shape of the feet (page 135) shows how well they are shaping up.
- The size of the feet (page 191) indicates how they size themselves and others up.
- Changes in skin colouring (page 93) that highlight surfacing emotions.
- Note the texture of the skin (page 40), as well as markings (page 107) and impressions (page 65).
- Pay attention to the state and condition of their nails (page 48).
- Gently hold their feet whilst doing this to gauge their temperament through the temperature.

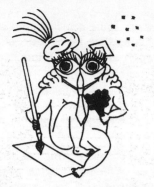

FEET SHOW HOW MULTI-TALENTED INDIVIDUALS ARE.

VISUALIZING THE BODY ON THE FEET

To really understand feet, visualize the body on them, in miniature, in the following way:

- the front of the body on the soles of the feet
- the back of the body on top of the feet
- the right half of the body on the right foot and the left half on the left foot
- the solidarity of the hips and pelvis on the firm heels
- the abdominal region on the fleshy insteps
- the bony ribcage on the balls of the feet
- the neck and throat on the toe necks
- the head on the toes.

The imagery tends to be a little more confusing when reaching the toes since the body only has one head with two sides, yet there are ten toes, with five on either foot. However, each set of toes reflects a specific aspect of the multidimensional mind, which helps in understanding how the individual thinks. Now visualize:

- the shoulder sockets reflexes (page 79), which are two tiny knobbly bones, just beneath the little toes, on top of the feet
- the elbow reflexes (page 150) being the small bones, halfway down the outer edges of both feet
- the two sides of the spinal column (page 55) along the bony arches
- the internal organs (page 160) on the fleshy parts just beneath the arches.

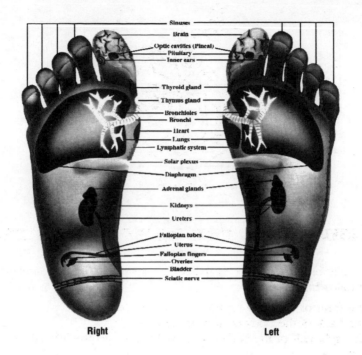

Right   Left

FEET ARE MICROCOSMS OF THE BODY.

Additional bones or extra organs, such as a third kidney, also show up on the feet, as do any missing organs or parts that have been removed. Significant changes of mind that affect the body alter the appearance of the corresponding reflex to highlight the issue.

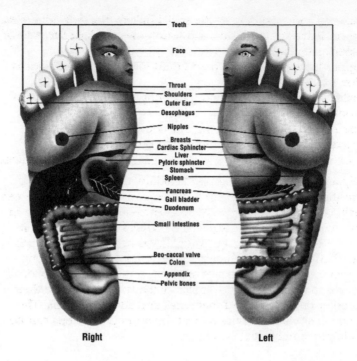

Teeth
Face
Throat
Shoulders
Outer Ear
Oesophagus
Nipples
Breasts
Cardiac Sphincter
Liver
Pyloric sphincter
Stomach
Spleen
Pancreas
Gall bladder
Duodenum
Small intestines
Beo-caccal valve
Colon
Appendix
Pelvic bones

Right   Left

WHEN THE BODY PLAYS UP, IT SHOWS IN THE FEET.

THE MEANINGS OF THE REFLEXES

Everything in life is meaningful and absolutely nothing happens by accident. It has to be this way otherwise there would be no order or no reason to live. Yet the rationale is not always obvious, which is why everybody is given the opportunity to work things out for themselves through their experiences and interactions with others. Anything that is contrary to their expectations is picked up by their feet, so knowing the significance and specific meaning of each reflex helps in interpreting what the message-laden feet are trying to convey.

- The heels and little toes talk of security and stability, along with the impetus and flexibility to get moving, depending on how the family

is structured and according to the social beliefs that they adhere to.
• The lower halves of the instep and fourth toes disclose the state of one's personal relationships.
• The upper halves of the instep and third toes reveal the ability to function efficiently and effectively.
• The balls of the feet and second toes bring to the fore feelings of self-worth and self-esteem.
• The toe necks let on whether the individual is speaking up for themselves or needlessly succumbing to others.
• The toes reveal how good the individual is at stretching their mind.

The body and feet naturally extrude health, with the only thing getting in their way being the mind. When a major issue is made out of something relatively unimportant, the internal havoc shows up in the relevant 'tissue', which is likely to be reflected onto the feet. In this way the 't-issue' mirrors 'the issue'. If, however, the situation is seen for what it is and that there is a reason for things happening then neither the body nor the feet are adversely affected. Individuals generally respond differently to similar circumstances because their agendas differ due to amassed memories and adopted beliefs. The feet change their characteristics so that the appropriate steps can be taken to improve unhealthy situations.

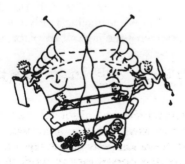

INSIGHT FROM THE FEET!

AT THE ROOT OF DISEASE

It's one thing to get the gist of what feet are trying to say, but it's another to try and find the solution. This, of course, is crucial if life circumstances are to improve, which is why it is so important to keep questioning to get to the root of any sickness, illness or disease. First find out when the symptom, or symptoms, began and then ask what was going on in their life at that time. Next, invite the individual to describe their symptoms so that they can be linked to an emotionally distraught memory. Those symptoms that started during childhood indicate that the mother, or surrogate parent, was going through a particularly unsettling time. So look at the symptom to determine what was afoot at that time.

- Aches indicate a deep need or complete dread of something important.
- Bleeding is an outpouring of extreme unhappiness, usually when there is little or no love, approval or recognition.
- A blister reveals friction in a sensitive area.
- A broken bone is a sign of needing to break free or make a break, yet reluctant or refusing to do so.
- Bruising typically comes from being really hurt about being taken advantage of, knocked about or constantly put down.
- A cut commonly occurs when feeling badly cut up or cut off.
- Dislocation is indicative of feeling out of place, not belonging or disconnected in some way.
- Hot flushes come from subconscious embarrassment or from getting hot under the collar.
- Infection is an outlet for intense fury, tremendous frustration or burning anger.
- Itching can be due to excessive irritability or great impatience.
- Numbness is a subconscious way of not feeling a memory from the past because of the pain it evokes.
- Paralysis generally comes from a paralyzing fear that brings things to a standstill.
- Sweating is usually a sign of being really uptight or anxious.

The body and feet swell to indicate a need for more space or when overwhelmed, whereas they sink or become flaccid when utterly exhausted or feeling deflated or deprived, or when denied something crucial. Once the bothersome source has been unearthed, the next step is to determine what can be done to make things better, which is best achieved through a small adjustment within the mind.

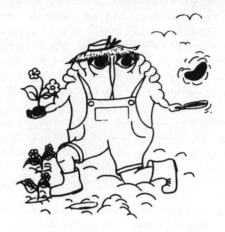

GETTING TO THE ROOT OF IT ALL!

02 On the toes!

OBSERVE THE TOES

It is fascinating to see how feet move during a heartfelt discussion or when in deep thought, with passion causing the toes to become highly animated, even whilst the rest of the body is still. Feet speak absolute volumes, especially through the movement of their toes, which is particularly obvious on babies and young children whose feet have much to say long before any words come out of their mouths. Youngster's toes spread with delight when alert and interested, whereas embarrassment or uncertainty causes their toes to bend over themselves and curl. Since children generally like to think for themselves, they tend to hate wearing shoes because it prevents them from doing so, which is also why free thinkers invariably prefer to go barefoot or slip their feet into a pair of open shoes so that their toes, along with their ideas, are free and open to the elements. Yet many highly-evolved teenagers bury their feet in the deep confines of heavy boots and lace-up shoes for fear of what would happen if their extraordinary ideas, which are way beyond most people's comprehension, came out into the open, yet these phenomenal concepts are so desperately needed for human evolution.

When feeling wobbly it's the toes that get a firm grip on things by folding mercilessly underneath themselves, particularly when extremely anxious or highly distressed. The subsequent pressure on the brain reflexes reveals a lack of space in which to think at times like these. Footwear (page 201) also tends to restrict natural movement and, when too tight, can cramp one's style, as individual views, as well as the toes, bend in a desperate attempt to fit in. With toes symbolizing structured thoughts and adopted belief systems, their small bones, known as the phalanges, are far stronger when the mind is filled with more substantial and meaningful thoughts, making it possible to think more coherently. Toes reveal whether the thoughts in mind are adequately supportive of one's personal needs.

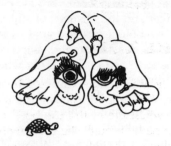

TOES REVEAL WHAT'S ON THE MIND.

NOTE

When writing an exam, giving a speech or during any stressful situation, it helps to open the toes and spread them as wide as possible, and keep them that way by placing them flat on the ground. It's amazing how this can increase confidence and enhance mental alertness.

WHATEVER IS ON THE MIND

Feet know everything there is to know about the mind, body and spirit, with each of their miniscule cells remembering every step that has ever been taken, along with the thoughts and feelings at the time. Those events that had the greatest impact on the soul invariably leave an impression or mark on the soles, which is why every step is subconsciously considered to be an asset or a hindrance. Even though the feet take the brunt for everything that happens, they are constantly prepared to take the next step unless the situation gets so painful or so bad that they have to bring things to a sudden standstill so that something is done to improve the situation. Whatever the mind decides, the feet make happen and continually follow through. Yet the mind is so multidimensional and full of mind chatter, that there is the tendency for thoughts to be everywhere, often making it difficult to focus on the present. Furthermore, heavy, burdensome thoughts not only make life heavy going but also increase the likelihood of swollen feet and the chances of stubbing a toe.

So, as toes reflect the content or discontent of the mind, they constantly change their shape, size, stature, skin condition or colouring to get the message across, especially when thoughts get in the way of progress. Whenever ongoing disharmony plays havoc in the mind and causes mayhem in the body, the feet, and especially the toes, are likely to become distorted. This is when a change of mind can help to make things so much better. Yet the general belief that the physical world and other people are responsible for all ills and misfortunes has lead to the misguided conclusion that solutions are only available in the physical world. Fortunately, this is now changing, with the realization that chemicals cannot cure emotional pain and surgery cannot remove deep hurts, although they can certainly ease them for a while. For healing to occur, and to prevent symptoms from reoccurring, there has to be a complete mind change. It's fearful and vindictive thoughts that cause an unbelievable amount of inner tension, destruction and confusion, whereas loving, kind thoughts immediately relax and harmonize the whole body so that the best possible health can be enjoyed.

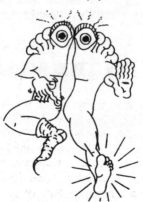

FEET KNOW WHEN SOMETHING'S WRONG.

TOES REVEAL INNERMOST THOUGHTS

Toes naturally balance the body whilst continually reaching out, like antennae, to seek new information, which is particularly necessary when venturing out and entering virgin territory. The toes also help determine the most beneficial steps when needing to move on; and when to stay on one's toes in readiness for anything that comes one's way. The following are useful guidelines in understanding how to assess toes and get an idea of what's going on.

- Each pair of toes symbolizes specific aspects of the mind.
- The toe pads reflect the face and reveal changes in attitude and the approach to life.
- Collectively and individually every toe has its own story to tell with each toe showing its particular slant on things.
- The right toes reveal past thoughts, whereas the left toes display current notions.
- The shapes (page 35) of the toe pads outline the frame of mind in which ideas take shape.
- Their statures (page 36) reveal the ability to stand up for oneself and face the world.
- The size (page 36) shows the amount of space in which to think.
- The direction (page 37) in which the toe pads face show the way one is headed.
- The colouring (page 93) and nature of the skin (page 40), as well as any markings (page 39) reveal the effect of the subconscious mind.
- The relative lengths (page 33) of each toe disclose the lengths one goes to express one's true self.
- The toe's flexibility indicates mental agility.

When first catching sight of toes, note your initial reaction and the words mentally used, since these bring to the fore what is subconsciously going on in the confines of the mind. For instance, toes that look strong and forceful could either reveal a deep thinker with intense or passionate views, or the desperate need to appear tough in the face of adversity. Meanwhile weak-looking toes could be due to extreme tiredness or a temporary lack of gumption in standing up for oneself. The unbending ways of society are at the root of extreme anger, fear and frustration. Contrary to belief, strict rules and regulations do not suit human nature and generally bring out the worst in individuals, which can be a bone of contention in later life. All is not lost though because this intense energy can be transformed into something really positive and helpful.

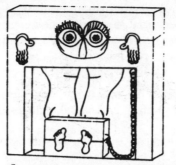

STRINGENT RULES RULE OUT LENIENCY.

THE INDIVIDUALITY OF EACH PAIR OF TOES

Each pair of toes reflects a specific aspect of the various realms of thought, giving them each a character of its own.

- **The big toes** are in the most powerful and influential position revealing core beliefs, intellectual notions and intuition.
- **The second toes,** with their air-like qualities, mirror the emotional aspects of thoughts that are needed to get a feel for life and to get in touch with oneself and others.
- **The third toes** rebound with ideas of what to do or not do; by keeping prior failures and successes in mind, which either dampen or fire enthusiasm and determine how the mind is made up.
- **The fourth toes** reveal inner mind chatter and the effect on relationships.
- **The little toes** reflect the embodiment of family's and society's belief systems and the impact of these on the true spirit of the individual.

Each set of toes also reveals the ability or inability to expand ideas beyond the norm and think for oneself, providing the foundation and stability to fully experience life.

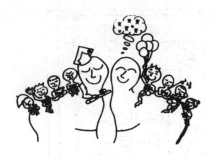

EACH TOE IS UNIQUE.

STRETCHING THE TOES

With some toes being long and pointed and others being short and
rounded, each toe has a character of its own. If they are consciously
stretched wide apart, it soon becomes obvious which toes pull away
from the soles, holding back ideas, and which toes push themselves
forwards, to get their point across, when the mind is stretched.
Meanwhile the openness of the toes reveal the openness of the mind
and the ability to embrace external thoughts. Those toes that pull away
from the soles highlight the notions that are kept to oneself and possibly
holding one back; whereas those that push forwards draw attention to
thoughts that are at the forefront of the mind. Toes that cannot separate
when stretched apart indicate a reluctance to relinquish control or hold
themselves together and form a united front no matter what.

Meanwhile, well-proportioned toes are a sign of a balanced and
well-adjusted mind, especially when their tops are all in a straight
line, confirming consistency of thought and ongoing level-
headedness. Unevenness in the heights of toes reveals unpredictability
and uncertainty, with thoughts being up in the air the one moment
and down in the dumps the next! The suppleness of toes reveals the
ability to adapt to new ways of thinking and the capacity to change
one's mind; although being too supple could mean that others are
tempted to take advantage. All of life experiences are coloured by
thought, so the colours (see Note on page 96) of the toes, especially
when stretched, can be very insightful. Although two individuals may
think the same and have similarly-shaped toes, their memories and
beliefs are likely to be different.

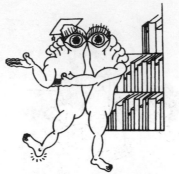

OPEN THE TOES TO OPEN THE MIND.

AS IDEAS TAKE SHAPE

Not only do thoughts shape and pattern the future but they also influence the shape of the toes. At birth, being naturally rounded, they provide plenty of space to explore and play around with ideas. Once conditioning begins, however, toes take on other shapes, especially when forced into confined ways of thinking, which is why certain toe shapes are believed to run in the family. Distorted toes come from distorting the mind to fit in with unsuitable belief systems or from being knocked out of shape when knocking or belittling one's own ideas. This situation can get worse with age, as old, crippling and set ways of thinking set in. Yet toes never lose their innate ability to change shape. With so many diverse thoughts in mind, the toes tend to take on various outlines, which are better understood in the context of past and present ways of thinking (page 126). The impact of each thought also alters and remodels the shape of feet accordingly; so, if ideas are constantly suppressed or crushed then the toes curl in a desperate attempt to hang on, causing much frustration and extreme insecurity. When looking at each toe describe it mentally to yourself and then ask questions using these descriptive words. For instance, if the toes look 'peculiar' then question what 'peculiar' means or whether there is anything 'peculiar' going on.

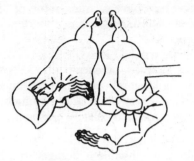

BASHING IDEAS DOESN'T REALLY HELP!

DIFFERING TOE CHARACTERISTICS

When a particular toe stands out from the rest, it determines certain types of thoughts, be them intellectual or emotional, that the individual is feeling. It may also be to do with activities, relationships or family. Relate this to what's going on in the individual's life. The right toes reflect past ways of thinking, whilst the left toes show the impact of current thoughts. Determine the various shapes as follows.

- Bent toes indicate difficulty in standing up for oneself, especially when there is or was no choice but to conform and be subservient.
- Boxed toes contain or box in ideas for fear of the consequences.
- Bulging toes reveal many ideas that need to be brought out into the open.
- Dented toes show that personal ideas are knocked because they are believed to be inadequate or ridiculous.
- An indented band around the tops of the toes that gives the tips a constrained, restricted appearance is from giving in to outside pressure, invariably leading to headaches and migraines.
- Pointed toes show a tendency to go straight to the point often with sharp, witty or hurtful comments.
- Rigid toes reveal uncertainty that can lead to obstinacy, strictness, severity or stinginess; a refusal to give into social pressure; a strength in standing one's ground.
- Toes shrivel or look insignificant when personal skills are not being used or when mentally drained.

- Solid, square-looking toes have a larger frame of reference and well-established ideas, although there is a tendency to be 'square' or old-fashioned at times.
- Squashed toes indicate crushed ideas.
- Straight, narrow toes indicate somebody who keeps to the straight and narrow way of thinking; who tends to be single-minded or have a one-track mind; who is very direct and extremely focused; and who is a quick thinker and immediately grasps the gist of things.

Toes get back into shape when the mind is filled with amazing concepts and something worthwhile is done with them.

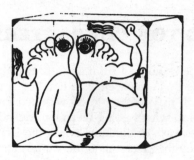

THE FRAME OF MIND DETERMINES THE SPACE IN WHICH TO THINK.

THE SIZE OF THE TOES

The size of the toes are a matter of personal opinion, with the individual deciding whether their toes are large, average or small. It's surprising how much perceptions differ since size is relative to one's way of thinking.

- Substantial toes are found on those who like to think things over.
- Toes enlarge when full of good ideas that don't always have an outlet or when personal notions are kept to oneself.
- Toes shrink with shyness, when there is little or no opportunity to think for oneself, or when terrified what others may say or think.
- Narrow, small toes reveal that there is no time and space in which to think or that there is no need to make such a big deal of everything.

- Smaller toes indicate somebody who belittles themselves and their unique way of thinking or someone who doesn't have to spend time on thinking things through.
- Streamlined toes belong to quick thinkers.

Ideally, toes should be nicely rounded and well proportioned, revealing ample space in which to think, daydream and play around with ideas. Being too rounded indicates that the individual thinks in a roundabout way, which is neither good nor bad, yet it can drive others crazy with frustration! The ability to think expansively ensures that life is lived to the full.

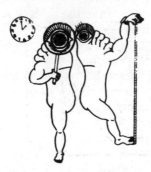

TOES REVEAL HOW THOUGHTS MEASURE UP.

THE INCLINATION OF TOES

The stature of each toe reveals the 'stat(e)-(yo)u-(a)re', which is influenced by the ability to stand up for oneself, especially when sharing unusual ideas and concepts in the face of adversity. Fearfully succumbing and bending into unreasonable social beliefs invariably has an unfavourable impact on the toes, forcing them to bow into submission and curl bashfully down towards the sole. Should the toes stand upright but slope off to either side, knocking, supporting or leaning on neighbouring toes, then look at the tops of the toes to see where the input of ideas is coming from. In other words, if the tops of the toes favour the right, then notions come from the past; whereas, if they veer to the left, then the mind constantly wanders into the future, sometimes making it difficult to focus on the present. The resultant insecurity can cause inflexibility in the toes.

- Toes knock one another when there is conflict in the mind.
- They support each another when additional inner strength is required.
- They overlap when the mind gets ahead of itself in one area and holds itself back in another.
- Toes bend:
  - from total submission
  - due to bending to unsuitable beliefs
  - when charging ahead with no time to think
  - from bowing down to please others
  - when curling up with embarrassment.
- Whenever a toe pulls up, away from the soles, it reveals:
  - a reluctance to get involved
  - stepping back for a while
  - not being prepared to step into line.
- Should any toe push itself forwards over the soles, it may be:
  - a means of getting one's own ideas across
  - a way of gaining recognition
  - a result of being in somebody's face.
- Toes become crooked from:
  - a constant change of mind in a desperate attempt to try and fit into unsuitable and unreasonable ways of thinking
  - devious thoughts and dishonest notions getting in the way.

There is less likelihood of matters becoming complicated and far greater clarity when the individual thinks on their toes with all their heart.

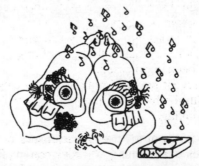

WAY-OUT THOUGHTS NEED TO STAND UP FOR THEMSELVES.

MARKS AND IMPRESSIONS

The toes often have tiny marks and indentations amidst a whole range of changing colours. These are particularly obvious at times of extreme vulnerability, since they are then more impressionable than usual.
To find out what these mean, describe them and ask questions so that their message can be interpreted, put into perspective and a solution found. Everything, be it a black mark, a white dot or a red blemish, is significant; since it highlights a memory or belief. Also every line is noteworthy because it too can provide some very useful insight when it comes to health and healing.

- Several horizontal lines across the tips of the toe imply an analytical mind that thinks step-by-step, being overly concerned and worried over little things that really do not matter.
- A vertical line down the toe pad, from top to bottom, may indicate a divided mind, seeing two sides to everything or a complete change of mind when, for instance, converting from one religion to another.
- Faint scattered lines usually reveal a scatterbrain whose thoughts are all over the place.
- A definite toe print discloses an individualist who is proud of their own unique way of thinking.
- A superimposed fingerprint indicates being under the influence of another.
- A long, hard ridge down the centre of the toe pad highlights the difficulty in bringing two very different ways of thinking together.
- An extra layer of skin that looks like a mask appears when putting on a brave face or when being two faced.
- Tiny pockets of what looks like a creamy substance, just beneath the skin's surface, indicate small collections of angry, infuriating thoughts that have been suppressed.
- Corns pop up to prevent personal notions from being trodden on or stamped out, with the hard skin preventing complete submission to other ways of thinking.

It's interesting to see how quickly the characteristics of the toes can change, with bent toes straightening, shy toes coming forward, angry-looking toes calming down and so on, any of which can happen as soon as there is a change in consciousness, which the toes immediately pick up and reflect.

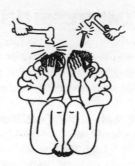

KNOCKING THOUGHTS MAKES IT DIFFICULT TO THINK STRAIGHT.

THE SKIN ON THE TOES

The skin on the toes is intentionally highly sensitive so that the horizon can be scanned at ground level for a quick reaction to whatever is in mind. The more emotive thoughts tend to get under the skin, whereas the texture reveals the 'text-(yo)u-(a)re', generally influenced by 'text' books studied at school. When the skin on the toes looks healthy, pliable yet firm, wholesome, balanced thoughts are in mind making it easier to deal with anything that comes to a head. However, as soon as thoughts are believed to be under attack then the skin thickens, particularly in the more vulnerable areas. Hard skin also acts as a buffer when, for whatever reason, innermost thoughts need concealing and kept to oneself. Hard skin obscures what is really on the mind and often makes it difficult to think straight. By constantly changing its appearance the skin gives vital clues of what is really going on beneath the surface. Some of the inconsistencies to look for include:

- Peeling skin arises when letting go of old ways of thinking and making way for exciting new ideas during times of transition or when there is a complete change of mind.
- The skin on the toes splits when mentally divided or pulled in many directions.
- Rough skin on the toes generally indicates a rough patch during which it is difficult to think.
- Tautness on the toes comes from extreme anxiety and concern or very set and rigid ways of thinking.

- Shiny toes are a sign of being constantly chaffed, trying to soothe things over or a light-bulb moment.
- A pitted appearance on the toes could be from knocking one's own notions or lacking belief in one's own way of thinking.
- A flattened toe pad is usually from falling flat on one's face or when the face is flat against the wall and there is a need get up really close and personal.
- A nice rounded toe pad, with nothing untoward marking it, has nothing to worry about except that life could seem a little bland at times.

Once the overall appearance of the toes has been figured out then visualize the face on the toe pads, with the right side on the right toe pads and the left side on the left toe pads. This helps to see how well the individual is facing up to their reality. When placed side by side, the combined outline of both big toes usually emulates the shape of the face.

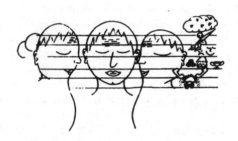

THE MULTIDIMENSIONAL MIND REFLECTS ITS MANY FACES.

ON TOP OF THE TOES

The tips of the toes reflect the top of the head and reveal the source of incoming ideas. They are energetically linked to the big toes and thumbs, as well as the toe necks and pituitary gland. When the toes are upright, there is a direct link to the Universal source of wisdom, but as soon as they lean to one side or another, there is much greater difficulty in thinking straight. Should the tops favour the right, then the information comes from the past, with the possibility of some ancient wisdom coming through; whilst a preference for the left indicates that the notions are way ahead of their time or there is a tendency to constantly plan ahead and live in the future. Look out for the following features:

- Hard skin over the tops of the toes could be a sign of:
  - intolerance, due to being a perfectionist, which is why other people's incompetence gets up the nose
  - finding it hard to get one's own ideas across
  - protecting one's real thoughts.
- Flaking skin on top of the toes reveals:
  - extreme irritability
  - total exasperation with other people's flaky approach getting on the nerves.
- Flaking skin over hard skin usually occurs when:
  - there is a high degree of irritability at having to conceal intense annoyance
  - experiencing extreme difficulty due to a constant change of mind.
- Initials, numbers or images often appear near or on top of the toes:
  - initials generally indicate something or somebody occupying the mind or an initial reaction to something important
  - a number could mean a number of things, such as counting the number of days to an exciting event or the number of things on one's mind
  - images take on a form of their own.

Take a closer look at the tips of the toes when there is extreme nervousness, endocrine (hormone) imbalance, oversensitivity or extreme insensitivity for clues as to what is going on in the deep subconscious. Should anything be amiss or unusual then check the big toes, as well as the toe necks, pituitary and thyroid gland reflexes, since these are all connected to the top of the head. Immediately beneath the tips of the toes are the temple and forehead reflexes, which mirror the way in which thoughts are processed. A furrowed brow is a sign of concern and worry, yet it becomes smooth when feeling unperturbed or reassured. Once the initial cause of any anxiety is unearthed, it is so much easier to know what to think to make things better.

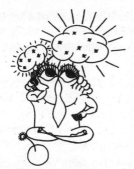

THINKING OFF THE TOP OF YOUR TOES.

A LOOK AT THE EYE REFLEXES

The slight mounds in the centres of each toe pad are the eye reflexes that reveal just how incredible the eyes are. They are a means of communicating with the rest of the world through images and visual impressions and, in so doing, provide a sense of space and proportion, from which various points of view and opinions can be formed. Meanwhile the mind's eye, otherwise known as the 'third eye', has the intuitive capacity to see beyond the obvious, as well as beyond the physical, which gives the foresight and vision needed for the gut feel for life. When the eyes are healthy, their reflexes appear well-balanced and vibrant. They, along with the pineal gland reflexes, are energetically linked to the second toes, index fingers and balls of the feet, and reveal innermost feelings and the true essence of the spirit. This is why they are called the 'windows to the soul' since they are also linked to the thymus gland, which is considered to be the 'seat of the soul'. The eyes, which are energetically linked to the second toes, as well as the balls of the feet, are in turn linked to the breath and heartfelt feelings. Visual difficulties may come from problems in these areas.

- Hard skin over these mounds displays momentary difficulty in seeing something that is vitally important, which fleetingly blocks intuition.
- A ridge of hard skin, down the centre of these reflexes, shows how hard it is to reveal one's true feelings, particularly when seeing things from two points of view that are worlds apart; which is why they are commonly found on visionaries or highly-spiritual souls.

- A line dividing the eye reflex reveals that feelings are only partially shared for fear of being hurt.
- A hard eye reflex indicates difficulty in seeing the trauma and sadness.
- Swollen eye reflexes could be from wishing to see more, putting on blinkers and turning a blind eye, or witnessing highly emotive incidences.
- The eye reflexes sink when tired of everything in sight or seeing things in the same old way time and time again.

Feeling sick at the sight of something or somebody comes from unpleasant and unhappy memories that can adversely affect vision. This can be remedied by focusing on the present and seeing the good in everything and everybody.

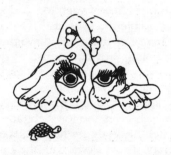

EYES FOCUS WHEREVER THE MIND IS.

A NOSE AT THE NOSE, CHEEK AND EAR REFLEXES

Immediately beneath the eye reflexes are the nose, cheek and ear reflexes, which reveal how ideas are interpreted based on memories of what happened or didn't happen in the past. It is these emotions that, along with current circumstances, determine the intent and amount of energy put into the next step. Meanwhile the nose, cheek and ear decipher smells, touch and sounds to satisfy the tendency to be inquisitive. They are energetically connected to the third toes and fingers, as well as the upper halves of the insteps, which reflect the liver, duodenum, stomach, spleen, pancreas and adrenal gland reflexes, all of which thrive on the success of one's accomplishments. These are used to re-energize the whole body. Everybody craves recognition for what they do so look out for the following features:

- An itch on the inner joints of the toes, over the nose reflexes, when itching for more praise, gratitude or respect.
- An itch on the outer joint, over the ear reflexes, from itching to hear more.
- Hard skin on the nose reflexes to:
  - stop the nose being boxed and put out of joint
  - show how hard it is to get the recognition that is craved.
- Hard skin over the ear reflexes reveal:
  - how difficult it is to hear what's going on
  - a reluctance to get involved with what's being said.
- A corn develops over the ear reflex when turning a deaf ear because of being too frightened of what may be heard since this could lead to inner conflict.
- Sinking occurs on the ear reflexes when not listening or when giving half an ear to all that is going on.
- Sinking occurs on the nose reflexes when the nose is put out of joint.
- Sinking occurs on the cheek reflexes from the cheek being knocked out of one.
- Nose, cheek and ear reflexes bulge when reaching out for approval and recognition or when needing more space to get on with things. (A bulging cheek reflex, for instance, comes from a deep need to be impudent and do something completely outrageous that could be frowned upon.)
- These reflexes may turn red when furious, embarrassed or frustrated by all that is going on, or not going on.
- Infection comes from utter infuriation and is more likely to occur on the ear reflex, which can develop a white corn, especially on the little toes, when furious at all that is heard within the family.

The ears and nose can and do change their size, shape and appearance throughout life, depending on how important the individual feels and their sense of achievement.

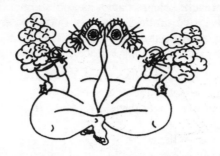

EARS HAVE THE CHEEK TO BELIEVE OTHERS; THE NOSE BELIEVES ITS OWNER!

TALK ABOUT THE MOUTH REFLEXES

The mouth reflexes are affected by what is said, which then determines the type of relationship that one has with oneself and others. They are energetically linked to the fourth toes and fingers, the lower halves of the insteps, as well as the ovarian reflexes. They react to all that is said and the decisions made, since chewing things over makes it easier to know what to take in and what to leave alone. The tongue, being the body's most powerful weapon, has the amazing capacity to strike out and give a nasty blow; or gently soothe things over. Whatever comes out of the mouth either enhances, destroys or makes no impact at all, so look out for the following features:

• Hard skin over these reflexes which may indicate:
  – difficulty in speaking up
  – fear of the backlash
  – a need to hold one's tongue.
• Flaking skin over the mouth reflexes appears when irritated at not having a say.
• These reflexes sink from keeping the mouth shut or from constant criticism.
• Mouth reflexes enlarge when needing to speak one's mind but not doing so or when forcing oneself not to say anything.

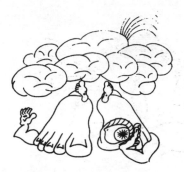

TIRED OF KEEPING THE MOUTH SHUT.

SIZING UP THE JAW REFLEXES

The jaw reflexes are firmly ensconced along the contours of the lower borders of the toe pads and reveal just how secure and set one is in one's own way of thinking. Greater security ensures greater flexibility, making the jaw reflexes appear relaxed and pliable. Their energetic connection to the little toes and fingers, as well as the heels, also links them to the pelvis, lower excretory and reproductive organs, especially the testes, along with the bones and muscles. These areas are all connected to the will, allowing the jaw to clench and unclench when thinking, which is why anxious notions cause these areas to tense, whilst free-flowing thoughts ensure far greater flexibility and mobility. When determined to get ahead the chin often juts out, which can make the jaw reflexes stand out. Should this go too far, then the obstinacy and stubbornness can bring things to a standstill.

- Hard skin on the jaw reflexes indicates:
  - extreme determination or inflexibility
  - an exceptionally strong will
  - self-justified obstinacy that others can find unreasonable.

Sometimes it is necessary to stick one's chin out to get ahead in life.

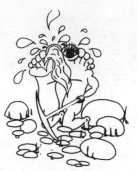

DETERMINED TO GET AHEAD.

ON TO THE TOENAILS

The horny coverings of the toenails reflect the skull whilst each toenail reveals just how much personal perceptions need protecting, especially when under threat. At birth, the cranial bones glide over one another, to allow the baby's head to adjust itself to the birth canal, and also so that the brain can expand as the baby starts thinking for itself. As the baby grows the bones knit together and ideas become set. A particular way of thinking may show up on the nails, especially when needing to be as tough as nails. Nails reveal what's going on at the back of the mind and help in getting to the root of profound issues.

Find out what the individual thinks of their toenails, whilst studying them one by one. Should there be problems with any of the toenails, check whether it is on the big toenail and make enquiries about their core beliefs; should it be the second toenail then ask about their innermost feelings, and so on. Also question what first comes to mind when the word 'toenail' is mentioned. Should there be a dislike of painted toenails, find out what or who comes to mind when the thought of 'painted nails' is mentioned and then check on the authenticity of that person or thing. Constant questioning not only uncovers what's going on beneath the surface, but also brings to the fore hurtful memories and damaging beliefs that now need to be put to bed. It's also useful to mentally describe the look of each toenail and be conscious of the words used, keeping the following in mind.

- Big toenails are generally larger since they safeguard mainstream notions, as well as spirituality; they are influenced by the state of the nerves, hormonal activity and the degree of sensitivity.
- The second toenails back up feelings and reveal the ability to breathe and circulate freely.
- Third toenails draw attention to the amount of backing available when putting one's own ideas into action and are also linked to the activity of the upper digestive tract.
- Fourth toenails hang onto the more intimate aspects of one's concepts and are connected to the lower digestive tract.
- The nails on the little toes may seem to be embarrassingly insignificant, but they do their best to shield and protect individuality within the family and society.

The characteristics of the nails are influenced by one's inner strength which affects the substance of the bones, as well as the strength of the muscles. They also rely on the willingness to let go of the old and make way for the new. Being punctual and staying on track avoids having to dig the nails in.

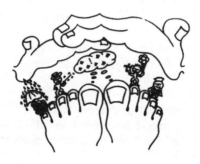

COVERING UP SOME AMAZING IDEAS!

HAVING AN IMPACT ON THE NAILS

The toenails, as the cranial reflexes, are excellent indicators of overall health, with any nail disorder or deformity indicating a lack of belief in one's own ideas. Nails can go to great lengths to cover up unique concepts and unusual ways of thinking, despite a deep desire to share them. Most nail issues stem from a 'I would if I could but I can't' type attitude, so it helps to get to the root of the dilemma to know how to sort things out, before having to fight tooth and nail to hang onto one's personal thoughts.

- Nails thicken when:
  - requiring extra protection
  - there are very set ways of thinking that give the impression of being as tough as nails.
- Ridges appear on the nails at times:
  - of extreme vulnerability and insecurity
  - when additional back up and inner strength are needed to get one's own ideas across
  - there is a resistance to a particular line of thought
  - when going against the grain and coming into conflict with the usual ways of thinking.
- Brittle or pitted toenails generally indicate:
  - an inadequate input of ideas
  - insufficient recognition
  - knocking oneself for not getting ahead.
- Nails split when:
  - undecided and pulled in many directions
  - divided in one's mind
  - wishing to break free from constantly having to please others
  - splitting hairs over something that's not really important.
- Toenails keep breaking due to:
  - a desire to break free
  - always having to be on the defensive.
- Ingrown toenails are found on mavericks who have difficulty in sharing their way-out ideas, so go to great pains to bury these incredible concepts.
- Toenails tear more easily when:
  - tearing ahead
  - pulling strips off oneself and others.
- Chewing or biting toenails, although seemingly impossible, is a sign of:
  - utter frustration
  - a biting concern regarding sarcastic and cruel remarks.
- Changes in the colour of the nail draws attention to surfacing emotions:
  - yellow toenails reveal feeling fed up at having to validate every thought and wishing to 'yell' and scream 'ow' because of being so frustrated

- bruised toenails come from deep hurt at being insulted or criticized, keeping sad thoughts to oneself or because of others treading on one's toes.
- Fungal infections show disgust at:
  - being taken advantage of
  - those things that eat away at the mind.
- Hanging nails hang around the edges and often get in the way especially when outrageous notions exceed boundaries.
- Toenails lift to reveal the impatience, intolerance or irritation that has been kept out of sight.
- Toenails fall off when it's pointless to hang on to old ways of thinking.
- Painful nails are a sign of feeling nailed and vulnerable.

Shorter toenails make it easier to stay in touch with what is going on deep inside or can be a sign of holding back or keeping a firm grip on things. Longer toenails either reach out or keep others at a distance.

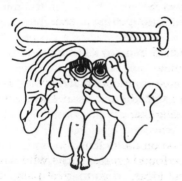

HAMMERING ONESELF HAMPERS PROGRESS.

NOTE

Toenails reveal pride in the way one thinks or shows whether the individual is putting on a pretence.

A REFLECTION OF INNERMOST THOUGHTS

Toes act as the body's antennae, spreading out and picking up on whatever is going on in the vicinity. Toes are so well tuned into every thought that they immediately detect the content or discontent of the mind, evoking deep emotions that then reverberate throughout the whole being. Toes reveal the profound effect that thoughts have on the body, with the most intense coming from angry, jealous, resentful and revengeful notions. As toes change their appearance, stance and stature, the sensory reflexes are shifted into unnatural positions, which distorts the way in which things are seen, heard, felt and said, to such an extent that it throws things off balance. This can cause deep insecurity within.

Headaches and migraines are also more likely because of all the painful and excruciating thoughts that are in the mind. To prevent the rebounding effect of all this, it helps to straighten those toes that have a mind of their own, which then makes it easier to think straight. Any thought, 'good' or 'bad', planted in the mind and nourished regularly invariably grows and develops, with the effect resonating according to its nature. For instance, tense thoughts tense the body; heavy thoughts weigh the body down and drain it of energy, whilst dark thoughts can lead to depression from constantly being in the dark. Detrimental and destructive thoughts may, in time, become toxic and cause sickness. The temptation to abandon one's mind and allow others to make decisions is appealing, especially when things go wrong, but it is so much more rewarding to use the opportunity to become better at being oneself. Thoughts are so potent that healthy thoughts can help to create a healthy life because when thoughts are good, life is good.

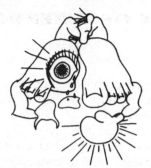

RIDDING ONESELF OF TIRESOME THOUGHTS.

SORTING THE MIND OUT

Everything in sight was once a thought! So, if things don't work out the first time, there is still room to change one's mind. One of the best ways to sort out the mind is to get 'organ-ized' so that the 'organs' and brain can function as they should. Having a straightforward, yet loving and honest, approach to life helps, although being too straight and going directly for the jugular can be crippling and bring things to a complete standstill. Good health is all about finding the balance between too much and too little. When harmful thoughts are replaced with loving joyful notions, things get to be so much more worthwhile, whilst freeing oneself from needless trivialities is one of the best gifts one can give oneself.

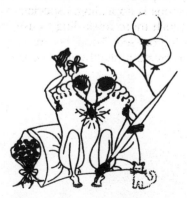

MAKING THE MOST OF EVERYTHING.

FIVE TOP TIPS

1 Let go of the past since it only holds you back.
2 Appreciate every experience for the expertise and knowledge it brings.
3 Constantly clear and change your mind for ongoing progress and fill it with thoughts that make you feel good.
4 Use free will to think in your own unique way.
5 Honour and respect amazing ideas and put them to good use.

03 The arches

STAYING UPRIGHT

The back remembers everything, including whatever has gone on or been put behind one's back, along with those people who the back has been turned on. It recalls times that the back was against the wall or when there was no backing and support. It carries details of everything that is subconsciously going on in the background, which forms the backdrop of life. These memories have a powerful impact on every step taken and determine how the mind is made up, which is why looking at the backbone reflexes, along the bony arches, helps to work out exactly what it is that is holding one back. It could be a backlog of data or a mountain of things that have been put on the back burner. These provide background information needed to determine where back problems stem from. The reflexes for the back have six distinct parts that stretch along the bony ridges of the arches:

1 The first sections, along the big toe necks (page 72), reflect the cervical vertebrae that show the amount of flexibility in expressing oneself.
2 Then along the inside edges of both balls of the feet (page 103), are the upper back reflexes where unresolved emotions accumulate, which, in extreme circumstances, can cause bunions.
3 Next, from the base of the balls of the feet to their waistlines, are the upper middle back reflexes (page 151) revealing the amount of backing and support when it comes to getting on and doing things.
4 At the waistlines of the feet are the middle back reflexes reflecting the point in the spine that, like the pivot in a seesaw, holds everything in the balance, which can get caught between what is desired and what is expected.
5 Then the lower middle back reflexes (page 167), between the waistlines of the feet and the junctions of the insteps and the heels, reveals the energy put into creativity and personal relationships.
6 Finally, sweeping underneath the inner ankle bones are the lower back reflexes (page 188) that show the type of basic support stemming from adopted family and social beliefs.

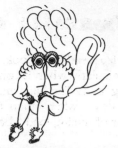

SUPPORT COMES FROM WITHIN.

With the spinal cord running from top to bottom, all the elements and colours are energetically represented in both arches:

- The ethereal aspect of indigo violet is connected to the big toes.
- The spacious air-like qualities of green run along the edges of the balls of the feet.
- The passion and fire of yellow extend to the waistlines of both feet.
- The fluidity of water and joy of orange flow from the waistlines to the start of the heels.
- The grounding effects of a deep earth-like red are found beneath the inner ankle bones to the tips of the heels.

Each element provides a completely different feel for the environment so that adaptations can be made for the back to be totally behind the body, especially when taking on something new. The back willingly provides all the strength and flexibility needed to go with the flow, whilst the spinal reflexes reveal the amount of inner dependability and reliability. For each new experience to be embraced, the backlog of memories needs to be released so that the back can be put into everything, making it so much easier to waltz through life.

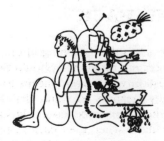

BRIDGING THE GAPS.

BACK TO WHAT'S REALLY GOING ON

Understanding back issues is like reading a book, with the back cover
giving a general synopsis, particularly when it comes to a bad back,
with the operative word being 'bad'. The back takes on dreadful
memories of being 'badly' let down when others backed out, of 'bad'
things going on back there, or of feeling 'bad' about going behind
another's back, and so on.

The back muscles are the first to put up a resistance whenever
anything goes wrong. It's here that piles of 'stuff' are dumped, to be
ignored or forgotten, yet it takes a lot for the back to complain. It's
only when it can't take any more that problems start! Being behind at
school or at work can soon build up and create a massive backlog,
with all the unresolved 'stuff' from the past being the last straw that
breaks the camel's back. The arches and spinal reflexes show that by
releasing the past, it's possible to step fully into the present.

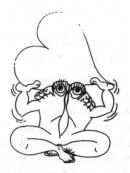

BACK ISSUES MAKE THE HEART SORE.

HOLDING ONE BACK

To determine exactly what it is that is getting in the way of progress
ask the individual to describe their arches. Should they use words
such as 'weak', then question what 'weak' means to them; or 'sadly
flat', then check what they mean by 'sad' and 'flat'. Listen carefully
since their words reveal how they subconsciously support and stand
up for themselves, particularly when their back is against the wall.
The amount of support the spine gives the body is closely linked to
the amount of support an individual gives themselves.

- Stiffness or pain along these bony ridges could be due to:
  - an unbending attitude
  - inadequate support
  - somebody in the background being an absolute pain!
- Arches tend to collapse:
  - when under pressure
  - after a crushing experience, such as a death, divorce or retrenchment.
- Arches that overextend may be due to:
  - stretching oneself to make ends meet
  - the strain of being a single parent
  - overextending oneself to support an elderly parent or a needy dependant.

Babies are generally born flat-footed due to being completely dependent on others to feed them, change them and carry them around. It's only when babies stand on their own two feet and start doing things for themselves that their insteps develop. The strong connection between the mother's and child's spines stems from the time in the womb, when the baby is completely aware of all that is going on in the background every time the mother thinks, feels or does something. The energy of the mother's more terrifying moments is stored in the baby's spine and can cause problems later in life, when similar incidences occur. Each third of the spinal reflex represents the three trimesters of the mother's pregnancy. They develop as indicated below providing that the mother isn't heavily reliant on others for support or is so highly privileged that she never has to lift a finger.

- **Top third.** The sections from the tips of the big toes to the bases of the balls of the feet indicate the amount of emotional support and encouragement the mother-to-be received during the first trimester.
- **Middle third.** These sections of both bony arches reveal the second trimester and the back up received during the second trimester.
- **Bottom third.** The sections that stretch beneath both ankle bones highlight the basic support, especially family and financial, during the last trimester.

Back issues date back to the mother's experiences during pregnancy, making it easier for a change of mind to improve the situation once the mother's painful and uncomfortable circumstances are understood.

The spinal reflexes bulge at times when additional support is utilized and collapse or become hollow when there is little or no support. Putting the mother's circumstances into context invariably provides the relief needed. By giving oneself and others backing and support collapsed arches and flat feet can be improved since the back up determines how well the arches are able to adapt.

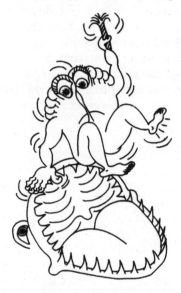

CONFRONTING THE PAST.

04 The big toes - the intellectual, intuitive toes

WHATEVER IS ON THE MIND

The big toes reflect masculine traits, along with the third and little toes since they are all odd numbers, which means that their approach to life is more direct and there has to be a good reason for everything. They, therefore, symbolize the intellect and determine the type of thoughts that constantly run through the body (either consciously, subconsciously or unconsciously), which are responsible for formulating the inner core. They are related to the thumbs, feet and hands, as well as the toe necks and their related parts. When looking at the big toes be conscious of what the number 'one' brings to mind and whether there is any correlation. If not, determine the changes needed to be number 'one' and find out how this could come about. Look to see whether the big toes look 'comfortable' or seem out of place and whether there is anything that is particularly striking about them to determine the impact of the core belief systems, which also influences the appearance of the inner edges of the feet.

The big toes resonate to ether and reflect the non-materialistic aspect of thoughts, then, at the same time, vibrate to white, indigo and violet which provide a direct link to Universal knowledge and wisdom. It's the faith and belief in oneself that strengthens the nerves, sharpens the senses and balances the hormones, all of which is mirrored in the big toes, where the main brain, sensory and endocrinal reflexes can be found. The sensory organs are constantly reaching out into the environment for sense to be made of what's going on in the vicinity so that the most appropriate responses can be decided upon. The big toes takes the lead in anything new, which is why out-dated beliefs and dreadful memories hold them back and are so 'bad' for the mind, body and soul. With around a quarter of the body above them, the big toes constantly strive to keep everything going, which is why they are known as the 'greater' or 'intellectual' toes, and are really big on openness, honesty and decency, as they show the way.

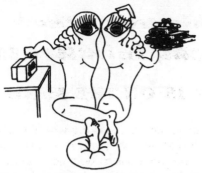

THE BIG TOES ARE AWARE OF EVERY THOUGHT.

IDEAS THAT LEAD THE WAY

The right big toe reveals past beliefs and notions, whilst the left big toe reflects the impact of current ways of thinking. Ideally both toes should be straight but supple, with enough flexibility to keep an open mind. Problems only arise when there is a resistance, or overly set ways of thinking, or when life is taken far too seriously. Fortunately a good sense of humour helps to balance the mind with the big toes following suit. Those who are confident, optimistic and independent thinkers usually have great-looking big toes; whilst highly-evolved individuals have longish, good-sized greater toes with oval-shaped pads, whereas those who are more down-to-earth tend to have shorter, stubbier big toes. The danger with the latter is that being too focused on the physical world can be detrimental to the true spirit.

The shapes of the toe pads on the big toes reveal the aptitude to think for oneself and open one's mind, whilst their sizes show the amount of space in which to think and play around with ideas. If they are too large, there's the temptation to procrastinate, but if they are too small then there may be a tendency to leap before taking time to think. When the big toes are much larger than the other toes, then there could be incredible thoughts in mind that are just too extraordinary and weird for others to contemplate, or perhaps the ideas are so visionary that there could be a reluctance to share them. Even though it can be rather daunting to be a visionary and a leader, the rewards are phenomenal. As soon as something really worthwhile is done with one's unique concepts, the mind can expand and the big toes can become increasingly flexible making it effortless to adapt to all the amazing opportunities that come their way.

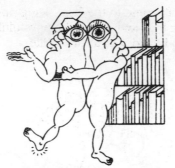

EVERYTHING HANGS IN THE BALANCE.

MENTAL CONFLICT

The big toes help the body to stand proudly upright but if one's own ideas are constantly shoved to one side, then these toes are likely to deflect from their natural course. This invariably causes them to change their appearance and puts pressure on the neighbouring toes. The extent to which these toes slant, reveals just how sidetracked the individual has become, especially when they lean on or bash the second toes, which then undermines self-confidence. Should the big toes totally obliterate the second toes, it is likely to be more difficult to get a feel for what's going on, as the emotions are being concealed. The more off-track the mind becomes the more likely it is for bunions to develop due to the awkwardness in continually accommodating other ways of thinking in favour of one's own. It is also easier to be thrown off balance, mentally, emotionally, spiritually and even physically, which may increase the need to control and be rigid. One of the main reasons for this is because of being totally dominated, overshadowed or subservient for a large portion of one's life, generally because of an exceptionally strict upbringing. Conversely, if the second toes overlap the big toes then the ego is likely to get the upper hand and undermine the logical thought processes, which can be extremely frustrating.

The big toes show the way, so when they saunter off into two different directions it is difficult to honour and fulfil one's soul purpose. Alternatively, if they are too stiff and point relentlessly ahead, it could be from the determination to get ahead no matter what, or utter obstinacy, which could develop into gout, should the arrogant, stubborn streak come to the fore. Being open-minded takes the pressure off the big toes and allows them to fulfil their obligation in getting the mind, body and soul ahead in life.

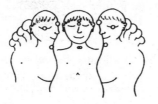

IT'S BEST TO MAKE UP ONE'S OWN MIND.

TIP

When standing with the heels together, the big toes should be comfortably aligned, to show unity in the mind. If they bend away from one another then it shows how far one goes to try and fit in or to be different or difficult. If the big toes are together for most of the way and then slant off at the joint, it reveals that one goes so far with one's own ideas but, at the last moment, veer off to please others or to soften the blow. To remedy this, separate the heels and place the big toes side by side; then, keep them together whilst easing the heels back towards one another. Keep repeating this as often as possible And, if needs be, place a piece of cotton wool or something comfortable between the big and second toes to get the big toes to stand up for themselves.

A CHANGE OF ATTITUDE

The characteristics of the big toes are affected by self-recognition and are either adversely or positively affected by the influence of dominant male figures. Constantly succumbing to incredible pressure or having things hammered into one's brain, can result in a hammertoe, whereas continually standing up for oneself in the face of authoritarian, dogmatic or brutish ways could cause the big toes to sink into their sockets. Getting too big for one's boots meanwhile, or getting in one's own way can increase the possibility of tripping over one's own two feet or of stubbing the big toe, both of which are harsh reminders that some gentleness and diplomacy skills would go a long way. To see whether one's approach to life is working well or not, look out for:

- A stubbed big toe which indicates that other people's ways of thinking are getting in the way or that one is trying too hard to be in control.
- Bleeding from any part of the big toes, showing an outpouring of unhappy thoughts.
- A bent big toe from bowing in humiliation, shame or submission, which is so contrary to their forthright nature.
- Big toes that withdraw or hold themselves back, away from the soles – a reflection of uncertainty, fearfulness, cautiousness or wanting to remain in the background.
- When the big toes push themselves forwards, over the soles, it could be a sign of trying to get one's views and opinions across to others.

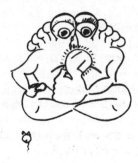

THE BIG TOES SHOW WHERE THE MIND IS HEADED.

HARDENED BIG TOES

Think of the three monkeys, who covered their eyes, ears and mouth so that they would 'see no evil, hear no evil or speak no evil'. When seeing hard skin on any of the toes, but especially the big toes, the sensory organ reflexes are affected and there may be difficulties with seeing, hearing or speaking. It may also thicken over ultra-sensitive areas.

• Along the tops of the toes to protect individual ideas from being beaten to a pulp.
• Over the eye reflexes, in the centre of the toe pads, when:
  – not wishing to see what is going on
  – turning a blind eye
  – refusing to see any other point of view
  – concealing or not trusting one's intuition.
• On top of the ear reflexes, on the outer joints, due to selectively choosing what is heard or turning a deaf ear due to highly emotive issues that conflict with personal ways of thinking.
• Over the nose reflexes, which are shared with the pituitary gland, on the inner joints, revealing the difficulty in getting recognition for hard work.
• Covering the mouth reflexes, just beneath the nose reflexes, because:
  – it's hard to keep the mouth shut
  – of the determination to stick to one's own decisions in the face of opposition.
• Bordering the jaw reflexes, along the lower edges of the toe pads, showing:
  – long-standing resentment
  – extreme anger
  – relentless determination
  – complete obstinacy
  – a suppressed need for revenge.
• Flaking skin over the hardened reflexes is a sign of extreme irritability at:
  – having to protect or conceal one's own ideas
  – feeling completely out of control
  – having to rely on others.

Other characteristic changes to look out for include:

• Swellings indicating the need to reach out to see, smell or hear more clearly.
• Unreal-looking big toes that look as though they have a film of plastic covering them and concealing the true identity; a 'Jekyll and Hyde' type of existence; a 'mask' over the whole pad from

putting on a front or being two-faced when it comes to sharing one's views.
- A superimposed thumb print on top of the big toe when under another's thumb.
- Markings, images, letters or numbers (see page 107), as well as colours (see page 93) also provide vital clues.

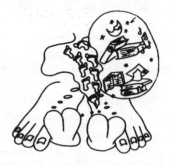

BEING IN TWO MINDS PROVIDES TWICE AS MANY CHOICES!

IMAGINING THINGS

Images are a vital link to the creative world and can be used to understand the true spirit. It is through imagination that inspiration comes, which then enhances intuition and provides greater insight into the inner self and whether life is working out the way it should. Images, symbols and ethnic signs appear more and more frequently on the feet, since they are an ideal way in which to convey vital messages and bring even greater comprehension of what is going on at soul level. Images show up on the feet as shadows, lines, darkened areas or glimmers of white, and are easier to see when your imagination is lively. Determine what the image looks like, whether it resembles an animal, person, tree, anchor, ship, fruit and so on, and then ask what it means to the individual concerned. Then formulate any further questions around their answer, to decipher the message and know what to do. The same applies to numbers, which stand for a number of things, such as the number of specific ideas in mind. Likewise for letters, which are usually initials of a person. Using the imagination expands the mind and enhances insight.

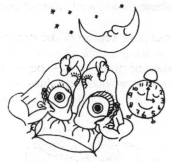

THE IMAGINATION OPENS ONE TO ENDLESS POSSIBILITIES.

TIP

Whenever an image doesn't look like anything in particular, draw it on a piece of paper and ask the individual what it means to them. If they have no idea, then suggest that, before falling asleep, they take another look at the image and place the piece of paper under their pillow to see what turns up in their dreams.

NOTE THE HAND AND FEET REFLEXES

The movements of both the hands and feet are influenced by whatever is on the mind, with the hands moulding ideas and doing something with them, whilst feet keep mind and body on the go, moving them from one experience to the next. The foot reflexes are miniscule but it is useful to know where they are. Their primary reflexes are in the centre, just above the bases of the heel pads, whilst their secondary reflexes are on either sides of the feet, beneath the outer ankle bones. Meanwhile the hand reflexes are often very prominent and often have masses to share. They are the slight mounds on the tops of the feet, immediately in front of the outer ankle bones. The right hand reflex reveals the effect of all that was handled in the past, whilst the left hand reflex shows how things are being dealt with now.

- The hand reflexes enlarge when:
  - losing one's grip
  - life is slipping through one's fingers
  - the hands are tied, making it difficult to handle things.
- Puffy hand reflexes indicate:
  - feeling overwhelmed by the pressures of work
  - contained anger and resentment at having to deal with a mound of unresolved emotion.
- Extreme tension in these reflexes comes from:
  - feeling uptight about one's dealings
  - gripping onto dear life
  - hanging onto something or somebody, who should have been released long ago
  - being tight-fisted
  - looking for a fight!
- Itchy hand reflexes indicate:
  - extreme impatience
  - a desperate need to handle things oneself.
- A superimposed thumbprint over the hand reflexes is usually a sign of:
  - being all thumbs when it comes to dealing with the finite details of life
  - being under another's thumb.
- Blue hand reflexes indicate:
  - deep hurt at having taken on more than can be handled
  - being upset at the criticism and judgement about the way in which situations are handled.
- Red hand reflexes reveal:
  - extreme anger and frustration at having had one's fingers burnt
  - humiliation of being twisted around another's fingers
  - infuriation of being at the beck and call of others.

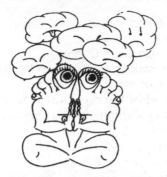

GIVE A HELPING HAND WHENEVER IT IS NEEDED.

STRAIGHTENING OUT THE MIND

Coasting along in a comfort zone stunts personal growth since doing the same old thing, time and time again, is neither stimulating or exciting enough for progress. The inner frustration can cause uneasiness which, in time, could show up as symptoms of disease. Yet the temptation to retreat back into 'comfort zones' is great because it seems easier to not to face or deal with disturbing issues. However, the memory still lingers at the back of the mind causing further uneasiness. Fortunately the big toes reveal any tension that is subconsciously building up long before it has a chance to develop into an unhealthy situation. These toes also reveal the effect of thoughts that constantly bounce back, showing why it is so important to think carefully before making one's mind up.

Wherever a thought goes the energy goes too, both externally and internally, which affects the chemical and physical content of the body and influences the characteristics of every cell. Thoughts, like pebbles dropping in a pool, have a ripple effect that either brings out the best or the worse or has little or no impact. As thoughts are constantly transmitted, they can be picked up and deciphered by anybody, which is why a change of mind goes such a long way! Everybody needs to be the change that they wish to see in others, because as one changes oneself others are inspired to do the same.

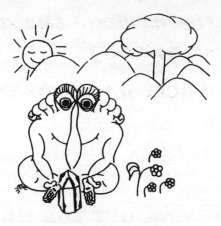

HEAVEN ON EARTH!

TIP

Everybody has a mind of their own, which when used lovingly and creatively is a great asset. The toes respond accordingly and will possibly even grow.

05 The toe necks – the ability to express oneself

THE RESOURCEFULNESS OF THE TOE NECKS

When examining the toe necks, look at their lengths on top and then underneath since the former shows the amount of talent that is inherent, whilst the latter reveals the amount being used, which is invariably significantly less. The longer the toe necks, the greater the imagination, which is why many musicians, artists, actors and fiction writers have such incredibly long toe necks. However, it is one thing to have the talent but another to put it to good use. Many of these highly artistic individuals have their heads in the clouds and have no idea, or can't be bothered, to bring these amazing concepts back to earth. Short, stubby toe necks don't mean a lack of talent, it's a sign of being more grounded and down to earth by nature. When it's difficult to see the toe necks because of the toes bending over them, then it's indicative of the difficulty in speaking up for oneself, which is why they are commonly seen on people who are forced to keep their traditions and views to themselves. However, there are those who have had words rammed down their throats or have allowed others speak on their behalf who also have insignificant or non-visible toe necks. So, look at the toe necks, especially on the big toes, to see how the authentic self could be brought out into the open.

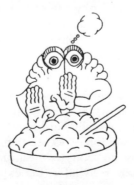

STICK THE NECK OUT AND PREVENT IT FROM WRINKLING!

THE ESSENCE OF IT ALL

The neck and throat provide space for non-physical thoughts to mingle with the physical elements of life as thoughts are put into action. In this way further ideas are generated and important decisions made as to the next step to take. The toe necks reveal the ease with which essential life forces are exchanged for ongoing well-being since the content or discontent of the mind has such a profound effect on the toe necks. This is why they give a good idea of how well the individual expresses themselves.

- The big toe necks show the willingness in sharing personal ideas.
- The second toe necks facilitate the two-way expression of feelings and emotions.
- The necks on the third toes reveal the exchange of thoughts when it comes to doing things.
- The fourth toe necks are connected to communications and relationships.
- The little toe necks are influenced by family and social beliefs.

Toe necks are constantly aware of what's going on in the head and thyroid gland, as well as the shoulders, wrists and ankles, all of which give the body the strength to believe in oneself and the flexibility to adapt to sudden changes that can then be taken in one's stride.

NOTE

The toe necks resonate to a mixture of ether and air, since it is here that the non-physical and physical energies combine. They also respond well to turquoise blue, the colour that connects the sky above with the waters below, although each toe neck also resonates to its own specific colour.

Difficulty in speaking up as a child can cause problems in expressing oneself later in life, especially when there is an intense need to always be 'right'. This makes it really hard to admit that others may have a valid suggestion. Being forced to see things from a parents' point of view leaves little or no room to speak up for oneself, causing an inner conflict that can adversely affect the expressive parts of the body and may lead to the individual feeling stifled or choked. However one must remember that it's impossible for everybody to see things from the same point of view; it's like looking at a house with some people viewing it from the back, others from the front and some from the inside.

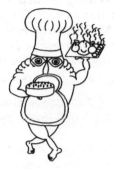

THE EXPRESSION OF INNERMOST TALENTS!

NOTE

Webs between the second and third toes are signs of a genius; not an easy role to play until it is acknowledged and embraced. Meanwhile webs on any of the other toes indicate that thoughts aren't compartmentalized, often making it difficult to be understood.

GETTING IT IN THE NECK

Thoughts that are allowed to flow freely automatically provide greater clarity, which helps circulation, particularly between the head and body. The livelier the mind the more nourishment and stimulation it requires, whereas loss of interest or fear immediately hampers the exchange of life force energies, causing the blood flow to become frighteningly diminished. Making matters worse are mental obstacles that are conjured up in the mind and build up in the head, getting in the way of the lymph flow between the head and body. This then makes it extremely difficult to let go of unnecessary thoughts that waste time and energy. The strain of this is likely to show up as wrinkles on the neck, as well as on the toe necks. Since the ears, nose and throat are so closely connected, any unhappiness from whatever is said or done could affect the throat reflexes. Most neck problems stem from the fear of being too open and voicing one's own opinions.

- Stiff toe necks reveal that tension has built up from:
  – not knowing which way to turn
  – a reluctance to turn one's head to get the bigger picture
  – very set ideas
  – being single-minded.
- Painful toe necks indicate that somebody is being a pain in the neck or is refusing to see any other points of view except their own.
- Lumps and bumps are common in the toe necks revealing accumulated emotion, generally from others jumping down one's throat or life being hard to swallow.
- Swellings on the inside edges of the toe necks reflect a lump in the throat from words being stilled, stifled or swallowed.
- Bulges on the outer edges are more likely to be the aftermath of disappointment, distress or grief, known as a post-nasal drip, which is a result of holding back or swallowing one's tears.

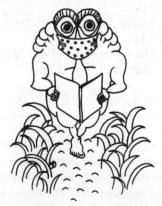

DRASTIC MEASURES TO KEEP THE PEACE.

COMPETING AGAINST ONE ANOTHER

These days there is so much competition as to who is best that any form of conflict invariably shows in the toe necks.

- Acne turns the neck red and boils down to:
  - being hot under the collar
  - fuming that others do not seem to care
  - frustrated that others don't even make an attempt to try to understand.
- Athlete's foot shows up when:
  - choked about a past situation that has become utterly intolerable
  - feeling downright rejected, overshadowed or repressed
  - highly ambitious
  - furious at being unfairly judged
  - frustrated at not being able to speak up.
- When the strain of it all gets under the skin then:
  - fungi flourishes due to being mercilessly taken advantage of
  - dryness occurs from being sapped of energy, making one quick to take offence and snap
  - inflammation stems from extreme infuriation and accumulated rage
  - weeping reveals that the toe necks are the only outlet for extreme misery and disheartenment.
- A straightforward skin infection in between the toes usually indicates intense infuriation.
- Chilblains are a sign of being scared stiff of saying what's on one's mind and what others may say.
- Corns crop up to:
  - save the neck after having the courage to stick it out
  - avoid being grabbed by the scruff of the neck and being manipulated
  - prevent getting it in the neck.
- A cut appears when feeling really cut up, cut off or wishing to cut away from all the nonsense but not sure how to go about it, such as:
  - from the concern of being in a cut-throat business
  - feeling that the head has been cut from the stomach
  - when there is difficulty in actualizing thoughts.
- A distressing split at the base of the toe necks, usually reveals:
  - being wrenched away suddenly

- a rift and great suffering
- feeling as though one's throat has been slit
- resisting the temptation to split on somebody
- a split within a relationship.

• Hairs, more commonly seen on the big toes, either protect or subconsciously pick up what is going on behinds one's back.

• Gangrene is a result of dark, deadly, morbid thoughts that consume the mind.

Even though society tries to clamp down and stop individuals from expressing their true thoughts and exceptional ideas, it is important to find ways to do so anyway, even though others may initially be upset. Few feel comfortable with the truth, especially when it hits a nerve, but it does release deep-seated issues that are far more detrimental inside the body than out in the open.

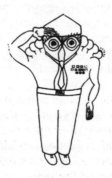

BRINGING THINGS TO A STANDSTILL.

THE LENGTHS THEY GO TO

The lengths of the toe necks show the lengths to which one will go to reveal what is really on one's mind. When the toes curl over their necks, it's to try to get a grip on things or to hang on for dear life, otherwise it could be from the embarrassment and shame at not being able to face others. Depending on how much of the lower surfaces of the toe necks are visible, look out for the following features:

• Lines on the toe necks due to:
  - feeling throttled

- the strain of trying to voice one's thoughts
- being fed up with having things thrust down one's throat
- swallowing unpalatable situations.
- Wrinkles reveal the conflict between the head and the heart, usually at the expense of the heart.
- Horizontal lines indicate:
  - where the line is drawn, especially when having to be restrained
  - the need to define everything
  - that words are having to be chosen with care.
- Two distinct lines keep whatever is taken in separate from whatever comes out. Since they are worlds apart, a vacuum is caused. This only makes sense to those who have these lines.
- A tense vertical strip stretching down the length of the toe neck reveals intense strain at having to swallow some extremely distasteful aspects of life.
- A hardened vertical ridge reveals the effort needed to compromise oneself, by saying what is expected instead of what one means.
- Patches of hard skin on the toe necks form over highly-sensitive parts, especially when feeling under attack.
- Scars are the remains of old emotional wounds that leave a deep impression.
- The appearance that a tight piece of string has been drawn around the throat occurs when feeling choked or throttled.
- A jester's collar along the base of the toe neck appears when constantly clowning around or having a wicked sense of humour.
- Flaking skin over the toe necks highlights extreme irritability from all that is said that goes against the grain.
- The colours of the toe necks highlight underlying emotions:
  - white toe necks are a sign of being tired of trying to speak up; completely exhausted at having to take in so much nonsense; or inspired to share divine knowledge
  - red toe necks act as a warning of being extremely frustrated; reveal intense anger; or indicate excessive energy
  - yellow toe necks hint at feeling really fed up or attempting to bring warmth into a cold situation
  - toe necks turn black and blue when deeply hurt and pained from getting it in the neck.

As alarming as all this may seem, it is all very manageable.

Reflexology is one of the ways in which to soothe the toe necks and ease deep hurt, embarrassment, shame, infuriation or divided loyalties. It's important for the authentic self to step forward and have a voice!

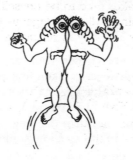

GOING OUT OF ONE'S WAY TO PLEASE OTHERS.

SPACE TO JUST BE

The thyroid gland gets it in the neck whenever there is a buildup of resentment from so much going on, making it impossible to know which way to turn. This is especially so after already having adapted and changed so many times to please others leaving little or no room to please oneself. The thyroid gland reflexes, perched on the inner edges of the baselines of the big toe necks, are so miniscule that they can barely be seen, unless they become noticeably enlarged. They reveal the amount of space needed to be oneself.

- The thyroid gland reflexes swell when:
  – constantly overwhelmed from doing so much for others
  – needing space to be oneself.
- They collapse when:
  – exceptionally tired of continually doing things for others
  – exhausted from trying to swim against the tide.
- Hard skin forms over these reflexes to reveal:
  – the difficulty in salvaging time for oneself
  – how hard it is to have a life free of constant interference and interruptions
  – the desperation in trying to protect the little time that one has.

• Red thyroid reflexes imply extreme anger due to
  – being in such a compromising position
  – pure frustration at never having one's own needs met.

Delegation of various tasks is one of the best way to solve thyroid
gland problems, since it makes time to be oneself. If this is not
possible then turning seemingly disadvantageous circumstances into
advantageous opportunities is a way of regaining self-respect.

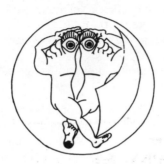

PUT ASIDE TIME TO JUST BE.

NOTICE THE SHOULDER REFLEXES

The slightly raised areas, immediately beneath the toe necks and
along the tops of the balls of the feet, are the shoulder reflexes that
reveal the 'shoulds' and 'should nots' in life. The right shoulder
develops problems from a righteous approach as to what should or
should not have happened in the past, usually because of a strict
upbringing or from taking on too much. The right shoulder is also
connected to masculinity, closely linking it to masculine-type
responsibilities. Meanwhile the left shoulder leans towards feminine-
type obligations and accountability in the here and now. Shoulder
issues occur when becoming too involved in things that are not one's
concern, yet they invariably prevent the free flow of life force
energies between the body and arms, making it difficult to move.
Look at these reflexes for the following indications.

• The number of swellings reveal how much has been needlessly
  taken on.

- Under the little toe: they are signs of unnecessary obligations to the family and society.
- Beneath the fourth toe: they are signs of burdensome and possibly heavy going relationships.
- Below the third toe: they are signs of unreasonable work loads that are not one's responsibility.
- Underneath the second toe: they are signs of a hefty out-dated emotional issue.

• The size of the shoulder reflex swellings reveals the immensity of that which has been taken on.

• Sunken reflexes indicate the exhaustion of carrying so much on one's shoulders.

• Hard skin conceals or draws attention to the difficulty of taking on so much.

By encouraging others to sort things out for themselves, everybody can get on with their own lives. Their capacity to do so is up to them; even if it means dumping stuff onto other willing shoulders. Freeing oneself of responsibilities is not a sign of not caring; on the contrary, it is indicative of caring enough to encourage others to do things for themselves. It certainly lifts a weight from the shoulders.

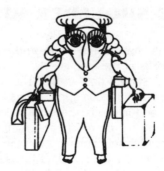

STOP TAKING ON SO MUCH FOR THE SHOULDERS' SAKE!

A GLIMPSE OF THE WRIST AND ANKLE REFLEXES

Life is a risk and risks are the best way in which to rediscover the authentic self and find out one's capabilities when push comes to shove. After all, there are no mistakes, only opportunities to try again. The wrists and ankles enable the body to make last-minute changes or bypass trouble spots. The only thing that gets in the way is the grudge of doing the same old thing time and time again, whilst the lack of variation stiffens the joints and causes rigidity.

The wrists are the bridges between thoughts and the ability to do something worthwhile with them, which is why problems arise when it's impossible to get one's own views across or when emotionally pulled in many directions. If this is really bad, then the conflict between what's happening and what *should* be happening puts tremendous strain on the wrists. Meanwhile the ankles are the bridges between the mind and the paths that one would like to walk. Despite their skinniness, they provide tremendous support and make sure that there is meaning and purpose to everything. Problems are due to a fear of stepping ahead, or of being rejected, or a lack of conviction, making it too terrifying to move. Taking a risk is the best way in which to break free from 'stuck' ways of thinking and 'stale' ways of behaving. Risks are the spice of life.

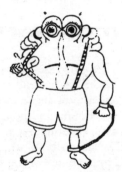

FREEING ONESELF OF UNREASONABLE SHACKLES.

TAKING A RISK

Not taking risks can results in a loss of self-respect. Even though everybody is unique, many conceal their eccentricities for fear of what others may think or say. Yet, this quirkiness is such an important part of being an individual and ensures that one stands out from the crowd. The continual pressure of trying to be socially acceptable causes a whole range of throat and neck disorders, especially when saying things to please others to the detriment of oneself. Attempting to fit into old ways of thinking deprives individuals of the opportunity to make a big difference, not only for themselves but for others, whilst suppression of the fun aspects prevents light-heartedness, which really isn't good for the heart. It's time to inspire others by being oneself and lightening up.

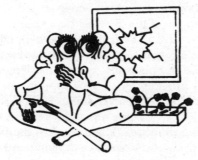

CHANGE TO PROGRESS!

CONNECTED TO THE SOLES

Toe necks show how ideas are processed and transformed into something meaningful and worthwhile, with the toes reflecting thoughts, whilst the soles reveal how these ideas are put into practice, generating further ideas. The coming and going of energy, from head to toe and vice versa, assists in determining whether certain notions are going to work out and what to do. As ideas are followed through then the overall shape and appearance of the feet could change. For instance, toes that are more dominant and overshadow the soles display an incredible capacity to think but a reluctance to do anything worthwhile with these notions. Conversely, insignificant toes with overly large soles reveal being on the go and possibly doing too much for others, leaving little or no time to think. Ideally the toes and soles should be proportionally balanced and complement one another.

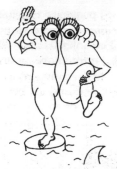

THE BALANCE BETWEEN BEING A THINKER AND A DOER.

FROM THE SOUL TO THE SOLES

Interestingly, the word 'sole' sounds just like 'soul', so it is hardly surprising that the soles show what the soul is going through. The sole's root-like connections link the soul to earth; because having the feet on the ground and the head in the air keeps the body and mind well balanced, whilst also maintaining contact with the divine aspects of the soul. With the soul being the vital link between heaven and earth, each sole takes it upon itself to reflect the impact of those experiences that have most impressed the soul. Being the whiteboard of the soul, the soles convey all that the soul feels, whilst allowing the soul to review and assess its situation before taking another step. The soul is the immaterial part of the body. It is believed to reside in the thymus gland, emitting moral and spiritual energy which forms the true essence of who and what one truly is. The heart gives the soul its spirit and brings the individual to life, its effervescence penetrates every single cell before radiating outwardly to form an extension of energy around the body, known as an aura. Although 'sole' means 'one', the two soles provide a balance, especially when the extremes are being tested so that life can be more fully appreciated.

Each sole takes on the 'opposame' characteristic of one's personality, namely:

- the right, reflects the yang and the left mirrors the ying
- the right, the male energy and the left, the female qualities
- the right, the positive aspects and the left, the negative traits
- the right, the enlightened energies and the left the unknown.

These are just a few of the 'opposames' that are at 'opposite' ends of the 'same' quality, thereby embodying the diverse nature of everything and everybody. The soles balance the extremes for a happy medium to be found. Furthermore an anagram of the word 'sole' is 'lose', which is why, when losing sight of one's soul purpose, it is so easy to lose one's way and end up being a lost soul. The messages on the soles of the feet provide guidance in getting back onto the feet and regaining a sense of purpose.

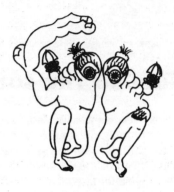

JOURNEYING ALONE, DESPITE BEING ALL-ONE.

TIP

Every experience sets the groundwork for personal well-being, which is why it is so important to understand where disturbing situations come from and to deal with the memory that evokes them so that the same old fearful pattern can be prevented from being repeated. The most effective way for an individual and their soul to evolve is by being an active participant in life, and by being completely present in each and every moment.

06 The second toes – filled with emotional notions

PUTTING OUT FEELERS

The second toes are two of a kind that emotionally balance the mind, body and soul revealing the more benevolent, empathetic and sympathetic aspects. The only way to get to know oneself is to get in touch with innermost feelings since it's the perception of oneself that influences self-esteem and self-worth. This, in turn, determines the emotional environment, as well as the ability to breathe and the condition of the heart. When feeling great it is so much easier to go with the flow and adapt spontaneously, but the moment anything gets on the nerves all this can change, making it difficult to get on and do things, even in the most conducive and loving environments. Being happy or sad immediately affects the composure of the body and feet, along with the energy flow to and from the second toes in particular. They resonate to turquoise green and air whilst their condition reveals the state of the heart and soul.

- The right second toe indicates past emotions, whilst the left second toe reflects current feelings.
- The lengths of the second toes show:
  - how far one goes to soothe things over
  - the natural capacity for personal success
  - the amount of influence that can be wielded over others.
- Should the second toes appear longer than the big toes:
  - first check that the big toes have not sunken into their sockets making the second toes look longer
  - genuinely longer second toes are known as Morton's toes and reveal the potential to be a leader, by example, due to having great vision and a tremendous capacity to feel
  - the ancient statues of the Greek goddesses are generally depicted with longer second toes, viewed by some to be a sign of extreme sensuality or athletic prowess.
- The shapes and sizes of the second toes:
  - provide insight into the ability to interact socially
  - show the capacity to adjust emotionally to unforeseen changes.

Feeling good fills the whole being with confidence and encourages the second toes to stand proudly upright.

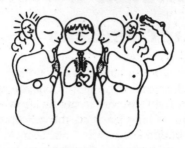

GETTING IN TOUCH WITH ONE'S OWN FEELINGS.

ABSOLUTELY DISTRAUGHT

The index finger is used to blame others or point out faults when feeling inadequate, yet this does little or nothing for the self-esteem. Signs that something is amiss include the following.

- The second toes stands back, away from the soles, because of:
  - needing to observe or survey the scene from a distance
  - wishing to avoid drawing attention to oneself
  - holding back personal feelings.
- The second toes pull away from the other toes and stand alone when:
  - believing oneself to be alone or isolated
  - trying to protect one's individuality
  - needing space to be oneself
  - feeling different from others and possibly unaccepted
  - feeling highly sensitive with the tendency to overreact.
- The second toes hide themselves away due to:
  - extreme shyness
  - wishing to keep innermost feelings to oneself
  - preferring to stay emotionally in the background or out of sight
  - the true personality being intentionally hidden.
- These toes look distorted or even have a false appearance when:
  - living a lie
  - not being true to oneself or others.

- They appear small and insignificant when:
  - lacking confidence
  - desperately needing love and attention
  - feeling overshadowed
  - emotionally smothered and stifled
  - constantly submissive
  - taking on the role of victim.
- Rigidity in the second toes comes from:
  - refusing to budge
  - being overly self-opinionated and dogmatic
  - a dreadful childhood with possible abuse
  - feeling like a nobody
  - being intensely passionate about something important.

Inadequacy and doubt can really knock the stuffing out of one, as well as cause the second toes to lean every which way but straight. Should the second toes overlap the third toes it could be due to:

- a fear of accepting responsibility for one's own actions
- feeling emotionally overwrought and not knowing what to do with oneself.

If the third toes prop up from the second toes it is from doing everything in one's power to hold oneself upright.

The more one resists terrifying emotions, the more they return to haunt one, until they are acknowledged, understood and released. When feelings are put to good use there is far greater confidence and the desire to become more of oneself.

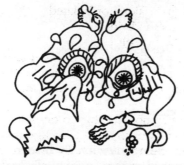

An OUTPOURING OF HEARTFELT FEELINGS.

TIP

When feeling unhappy or frustrated about not being able to air one's views then baring the feet and putting them up exposes the second toes to the elements and allows them to scan the horizon for a better feel of what is really going on.

SECOND IN LINE

The second toes have difficulty in standing up when there is a lack of belief in oneself, and it's the views that one has about oneself and others that influences their overall appearance.

- Bent second toes indicate:
  - the inability to hold the head up
  - extreme self-consciousness
  - curling with embarrassment
  - not wishing to get emotionally involved
  - being subservient and stooping so low that the toes look as though they are bowing
  - a massive emotional blow that flattens one.
- The second toe twists when:
  - emotionally pulled in many different directions
  - not knowing which way to turn.
- These toes bulge and look knobbly when desperately trying to find an outlet for pent-up feelings.
- Battered second toes come from knocking oneself for not being good enough.
- Second toes look squashed when pressurized by the big toes on the one side and bulldozed by the third toes on the other side, revealing:
  - a lack of space, making it hard to think for oneself
  - dodging an important issue
  - being bullied, burdened or hassled.

Feeling inadequate or constantly sorry for oneself makes the second toes exceptionally impressionable and pathetic looking. The friction in the mind wears away the sides of these toes, making them indented and smooth. If it's on the big toe side then there's a constant intellectual debate revolving around one's emotions; whereas, on the third toe side, it's likely to be an ongoing conflict about what one feels like or doesn't feel like doing. The shapes of the second toe pads reveal how those thoughts, that affect innermost sensations, take shape.

• Flat-topped second toes indicate somebody with strong intuitive abilities, which is why they are common on dreamers, artists, psychics, musicians, as well as some natural health practitioners.
• Hard ridges down the centres of these toes show:
  – how hard it is to look deep inside oneself
  – divided loyalties with the ability to see both points of view.
• Pointed second toes are found on those who:
  – go straight to the point when sharing their emotions
  – feel pressurized from both sides
  – suppress and fail to acknowledge their true feelings
  – question 'what's the point anyway?'

Truly believing in oneself and understanding one's innermost feelings goes a long way in getting better at being oneself. This not only boosts self confidence, but also enhances the immune system.

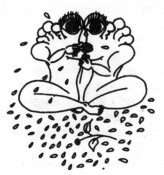

A HIGHLY SENSITIVE SOUL.

TIP

Stretching and straightening the second toes, with the feet flat on the ground, helps to get in touch with innermost feelings and put things into perspective.

SKIN CHARACTERISTICS

Feelings stem from thoughts, with the more irritating notions worming their way under the skin and getting on the nerves. With the skin being the largest organ of the body, its main purpose is to hold things together, yet it is more commonly used to cover up or camouflage true feelings. The body allows this to happen for a while, but should these start getting in the way then the feet will show how 'bad' the exasperating situation has become. Occasionally the feet may mask the true feelings, but they can be coaxed into revealing what's really going on at a deeper level. They do this by changing their colour, texture or condition, according to the mood, as well as all that is consciously, unconsciously and subconsciously in the mind. Whatever is being felt on the inside is generally reflected onto the outside, especially when it is an issue. Skin attracts attention to the unpleasant effects of horrible thoughts, ugly feelings and hideous emotions that have been shoved out of sight because of the frightful memories attached to them. They continue to do so until everything is sorted out in the mind. Feet are great at pinpointing the issue, enabling the ideal solution to be found.

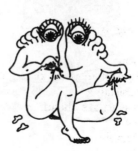

TUCKED UNDER THE SKIN.

Getting under the skin

The greater the concern about other people's opinions, the more sensitive and impressionable the skin. The skin reveals extreme insecurity and uncertainty, which is why certain individuals loathe being touched.

- Ticklish soles are:
  - highly sensitive souls
  - extremely self-conscious.
- Itchy feet indicate:
  - the need to make a change
  - wishing to get a move on
  - a desire for current circumstances to improve.
- Peeling skin reveals:
  - personal transformation
  - ridding the self of the old to make way for the new.
- The whole sole can come away in one complete piece:
  - during very distressing periods that are alien to one's nature
  - when wishing to completely tear away and forget the past.
- Extra layers of skin build up on the feet due to:
  - feeling vulnerable
  - needing a boost
  - hiding innermost thoughts and feelings.
- The skin hardens:
  - as a form of protection
  - to draw attention to problematic or difficult areas
  - when putting up a resistance
  - to show how hard it is to get ahead.
- Being too soft indicates:
  - feeling too impressionable
  - giving in far too easily under pressure.
- Flaky skin occurs when:
  - highly irritated
  - the approach is a bit too flaky.
- Flaky skin over hard skin highlights extreme annoyance at having to put up with so much insensitivity.
- Corns are also a form of protection; on the second toes they stop others from taking the wind from one's sails.

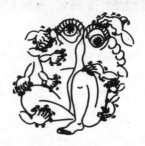

IRRITABILITIES THAT GET UNDER THE SKIN.

RUBBED UP THE WRONG WAY

Emotional wear and tear causes the skin to look lifeless and can make it ultra-sensitive and prone to extreme irritability. When there is a lack of understanding or things go against the grain then the skin is likely to change its characteristics.

- Shiny skin is usually caused by being rubbed up the wrong way.
- Blisters develop:
  - to highlight conflict in a specific area
  - to reveal emotional friction
  - as a result of ongoing resistance.
- A blood blister brings to the surface extreme unhappiness.
- Unusually smooth skin is a sign of:
  - having to soothe things over
  - a smooth talker
  - extreme difficulty in leaving a lasting impression
  - things constantly slipping away.
- Skin breaks out into a sweat when things are taken to heart.
- It wrinkles and becomes lined through constant concern or anxiety.
- It weeps with extreme sadness.
- The skin can become unpleasantly clammy when in a sticky situation.

Smelly feet usually indicate:

  - a life that stinks
  - utter disgust or extreme displeasure about what's going on.

- The skin splits when torn apart.
- It cracks when:
  - cracking up
  - feeling divided
  - pulled apart.
- Cuts appear when totally cut up.
- Bleeding is a sign of deep sadness usually because of a split or division.
- Plantar warts rear their ugly heads when feeling ugly about something due to much criticism and discontentment, causing a lot of frustrations, especially when feeling taken advantage of.

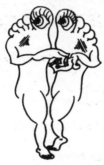

EMBARRASSED AND SELF-CONSCIOUS.

THE COLOUR OF THE SKIN

Feet constantly change colour to highlight emotions, with a more vibrantly coloured skin revealing a healthy confidence. The skin reveals the ability to blend into varying emotional environments and also brings to the surface prevalent moods that affect heartfelt feelings. Colour is strongly linked to memories and the sight of colours can stir a conglomeration of emotions, so much so that the skin on the feet often has a blotchy or mosaic effect. The patchwork appearance comes from a host of different feelings that overlap one another and reveal the type of reaction that erupts when under duress. Scrunching the feet as tightly as possible and then stretching them wide apart brings to the surface patches of creamy white or yellow, which not only reveals where the most disturbing memories

★ 93

are stored but also gives useful insight as to what the individual can do before the memories become troublesome or even noxious.

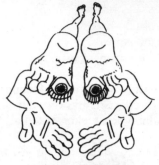

TRYING TO BLEND IN.

VARIOUS HUES

Every colour resonates to specific level of consciousness and is linked to a particular type of emotion.

- White is the epitome of all colours and shows up on the feet:
  - to indicate purity or divine guidance
  - to reveal utter exhaustion when totally drained of energy
  - as a sign of extreme fear or exceptional concern.
- Feet turn purple when:
  - spiritually aware
  - deeply hurt at being cruelly rejected.
- Bluish purple on the feet is a result of feeling highly offended:
  - on the big toes and toe necks – intellectual displeasure
  - on the second toes and balls of the feet – a battered ego
  - on the third toes and upper halves of the insteps – the result of injured pride or a disappointing failure
  - on the fourth toes and lower halves of the insteps – upset at being misunderstood
  - on the little toes and heels – deep discontent within the family and society.
- Black marks indicate:
  - deep emotional scars, often due to prejudice or non-acceptance
  - depression from being in the dark and not knowing what on earth to think

- morbid thoughts that darken the mind and drain the extremities, which can even result in gangrene.
- Green on the feet shows:
  - extreme discontent
  - a hint of envy
  - feeling dissatisfied
  - a good heart.
- Yellow tinges the skin when:
  - extremely disappointed
  - exceptionally critical
  - having a jaundiced outlook
  - overly enthusiastic.
- Patches of creamy, yellowish white appear just beneath the skin to reveal contained frustration, resentment and anger.
- Orange on the feet comes from feeling:
  - very unhappy at not being able to speak up for oneself
  - overjoyed at the pleasure derived from one's relationships.
- Red appears on the feet to show:
  - extreme embarrassment
  - total frustration
  - burning issues highlighted by sunburn or sunstroke
  - infuriating memories that continue to smoulder
  - intense passion.
- Feet are brown when:
  - feeling really browned off
  - trying to be more grounded
  - being involved in or affected by some dirty business.

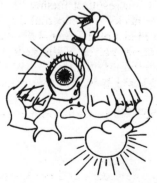

A COLOURFUL DISPLAY OF EMOTIONS.

NOTE

Autistic or mentally-challenged individuals often have remarkably bland and often unblemished feet since they tend to withdraw into themselves and mask their true feelings. Massaging their feet, with dolphin music playing in the background, gives them the confidence to start relating to those around them in their own charming way. Meanwhile reflexology also helps their parents and loved ones to adapt and be more accepting of these special souls, as well as help them to relate to their incredible intuition.

A CLOSER LOOK AT EYES

The eyes (page 43) are highly sensitive organs filled with emotion, so much so that they either bring a sparkle or tear to the eye. Their reflexes, on the central mounds of all toe pads, draw attention to the impact of innermost emotions. These are often remnants of terrifying, fearful or distressing scenes that were witnessed in the past and still need to be seen to through a more understanding set of lenses.

Since eyes are the windows to the soul, they constantly absorb colour into the body, even when they are closed. They help to throw light onto any emotional situation, whilst, at the same time, energizing the effervescence of the spirit. The extent to which mind, body and soul come to life depends on the content or discontent of all that is in sight and the perceptions and opinions formed. The eye reflexes are energetically connected to the second toes and the balls of the feet, which helps when it comes to determining the type of emotion that gets in the way of seeing more clearly. When toes curl and bend over themselves, the eye reflexes disappear from sight, revealing a poor opinion of oneself and making it really difficult to see the bigger picture. Insight gained through the eyes assists in working out the next step. Making the most of life helps in attaining a better outlook and in seeing things more clearly.

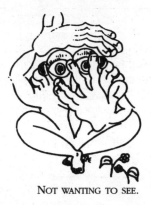

NOT WANTING TO SEE.

THE ONGOING CYCLES OF LIFE

The miniscule pineal gland is physically closer to the pituitary gland, yet is more influenced by the impact that emotions have on eyes. This is because the pineal gland functions according to the amount of light entering the body through the eyes, which is why it needs them to be clear and healthy. The melatonin that is produced balances the body's cycles and equalizes excessive mood swings. Any emotional disturbance or upset blurs the vision and throws the 'body clock' out of sync, whilst any form of negativity, be it anger, fear, greed, unhappiness or disinterest can cloud the outlook and interfere with the natural rhythms of the body. So it is that a lack of vision, not wanting to see, narrow-mindedness or being overly self-opinionated forces the intuition to take a back seat. This can adversely affect the tempo of the body, so much so that the blood circulation, as well as the lymphatic flow plus various bodily cycles, are easily upset. The mounds in the centres of the toe pads reveal the underlying emotion that causes this inner turmoil.

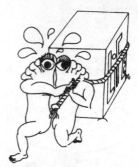

Hanging on to the past.

THE ANGLE OF THE FEET

There are times in one's life when it is difficult to know which way to turn, especially when there seems to be no point in going on. This is where feet can be really useful in showing the way since they point in the direction that the mind is headed. Being way off track is hazardous to personal well-being, because veering away from the centre causes the weight of the body, along with any hefty thoughts and burdensome emotions, to become unevenly distributed, causing awkwardness and discomfort. This forces the toes to cling on for dear life, putting additional pressure onto the eye reflexes. Furthermore the tripod, formed by the big toes, little toes and heels, provides the base upon which opinions are formed, with the second, third and fourth toes putting out feelers to get a better idea of what is going on. Any changes in this can adversely affect the inclination to get on. Feet are rarely still for any length of time and are constantly on the move, albeit very subtly at times. They have great difficulty in staying put, especially when the mind is busy, which puts the eye reflexes in many different positions as they subconsciously scan the horizon to see every point of view. Also note the following nuances.

- Pigeon-toed feet indicating:
  - innate shyness
  - an extreme lack of confidence
  - desperate self-consciousness
  - a sense of insecurity
  - a desire to keep oneself to oneself
  - a subconscious way of cutting oneself off.

• Feet tend to turn outwards when:
  – playing the fool
  – trying to attract attention
  – being too accommodating
  – way off track causing frustration, bewilderment or confusion.

The degree to which feet turn in or out shows just how far the individual has wandered from their soul purpose, which invariably affects one's views on life.

• Going on tiptoes is a way of:
  – seeing more
  – not wanting to draw attention to one's presence by being as quiet as possible.

Running to get ahead of the game is very different to running away, running wild or running around in circles, and whilst skipping for joy is one thing, skipping class is another ball game completely. Ensuring that the feet are parallel when walking helps point one in the best direction.

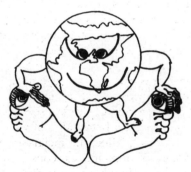

LOOK AT EVERY POINT OF VIEW.

TIP

To re-energize the whole body, stand with the feet parallel, toes wide apart, shoulders back and stomach sucked in. Take in some really deep and meaningful breaths that are full of white light and pure love.

THE TOE-HEEL STRIKE

When on the move, the toe–heel strike is influenced by the position of weighty thoughts and hefty emotions, since tension alters the stance of the feet. Meanwhile contracted muscles change the shape and size and, therefore, the amount of contact with the ground. When it comes to standing this depends on one's perceived status in life, with any shifting from one foot to another unconsciously realigning both sides of the body so that they both get a feel for what's afoot. The only way to completely still the mind, body and feet is by being totally in the moment or by being on one's best behaviour or under orders to stand to attention.

The gap between the feet, when standing, reveals the openness of the mind. If they are too far apart then others may be tempted to take advantage; however, this is also the ideal stance in which to give birth to new concepts and to be more receptive to new ideas. Meanwhile, anybody within the radius of the feet when standing and talking are those who are currently the focus of attention, although this can change as soon as anybody else comes along who wishes to be included.

Feet are often tucked underneath the body to get more comfortable or settle into oneself; or when feeling vulnerable or under attack. If placed under the chair when sitting, it could be from holding back and not wanting to get involved, or because of keeping oneself to oneself; or it could be a way of scanning the past. Alternatively feet stretched out in front of the body are a sign of feeling good about oneself or a need to get out there and be noticed, or it could be a way of stretching the point or getting more involved. Meanwhile crossing the left leg over the right leg helps seek comfort from the past, whilst the other way provides a glimpse into the future. Feet respond to the workings of the conscious mind when awake and tune into the subconscious or unconscious minds when very relaxed or asleep. It doesn't take long for the feet to realign themselves on waking, which means they become immediately aware of the nature of their surroundings.

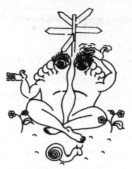

LIFE IS FULL OF CHOICES.

TIP

For some deep soul searching, close the eyes and place the soles together whilst breathing deeply and slowly.

IN THE PRONE POSITION

When lying on one's back the feet should look balanced and stand proudly upright since this puts them in the ideal position to re-energize and recharge the whole body, mind and spirit. As soon as the mind drifts into the past, the tops of the toes meander over to the right; whilst the moment thoughts wander into the future, then the toes lean to the left.

- Feet flop to either side when lying flat on the back:
  - due to exhaustion
  - when completely letting go
  - from being totally weighed down.
- Feet pull up, towards the body, because of:
  - holding back
  - not wanting to deal with something important
  - preferring not to get involved.
- Feet flop forwards, away from the body, due to:
  - a lack of strength
  - not being able to face what's going on
  - projecting the mind into the future.

- Feet bow over themselves, with little or no support from the arches, when:
  - the stuffing is knocked out of one
  - utterly overwhelmed or subservient.
- Bunions often pull the feet inwards, dragging the balls of the feet along with them, when in a fraught and often uncomfortable, emotional environment.
- If one leg appears shorter than the other, then it could be:
  - unconsciously holding oneself back
  - retreating into one's shell
  - not wishing to draw attention to oneself.

If on the right, it is related to the past, and, if on the left, it is the present.

- One foot pushes itself forwards when:
  - wishing to be noticed and seeking attention
  - being overly persistent
  - constantly putting the foot down.

If on the right foot the situation was in the past, and, if on the left, it is applicable to the present.

- Soles turn away from one another:
  - to avoid confrontation or inner conflict
  - when lacking the guts to deal with something important.
- Soles turn inwards and face one another when:
  - needing time for some introspection, especially when uncertain, unstable or depressed
  - confidence isn't too great
  - living in a world of one's own
  - mentally removing oneself from the demands and expectations of an intolerant society.

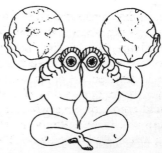

NOBODY NEEDS TO CARRY THE WEIGHT OF THE WORLD.

ON THE BALLS OF THE FEET

The balls of the feet take on the bulk of the body, as well as some of the more hefty emotions, whilst, at the same time, revealing the amount of self-esteem that comes from feelings towards oneself and others. This, in turn, affects the breathing. The subsequent buoyancy can be detected on the balls of the feet, along with the following.

- The respiratory tract reflexes fill the balls of the feet, showing just how one feels about oneself and others.
- The breast reflexes overlap the respiratory reflexes, exposing the amount of inner sustenance and appreciation.
- The heart reflexes, where the balls and insteps meet on the inner edges, reveal heartfelt feelings.
- The windpipe and oesophagus reflexes, along the inner edges, display the intake of new experiences.
- The thymus gland reflexes, midway down the inside edges, disclose the essence of the spirit.
- The upper back reflexes, along the bony ridges of the arches, divulge the amount of emotional backing that is perceivably available.
- The upper arms reflexes hug the outer edges of the balls of the feet reflecting the ability to embrace life.
- The diaphragm reflexes, along the domed-shaped bases of the balls of the feet, highlight the integration of feelings based on personal experience.
- The solar plexus reflexes have their true reflexes in the same position as the heart reflexes, yet are best detected in the central hollows of both feet. As the 'abdominal brain' it relays emotions to the digestive system.

The solar plexus is a highly emotional part of the body, connected to the element of air, which physically, emotionally and spiritually links the soul to its surroundings. This is why the impact of any interaction, through the breath or speech, can have such a profound effect on it and the digestive track. Any release of air from the body, either from the mouth or the anus, is the body's way of getting rid of stale air since it is full of rancid emotions. Overwhelming emotions not only hamper the breath but also distress the heart, which then saddens the whole body, causing instability in the blood. The balls of the feet reveal what is being kept close to the chest, whilst providing a firm, pliable platform from which the individual can interact with the outside world.

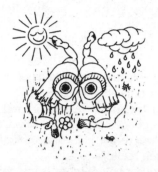

FEELINGS CREATE THE EMOTIONAL ENVIRONMENT.

HARD TO SHOW INNERMOST FEELINGS

It's really hard to breathe when emotionally distraught, which can, metaphorically speaking, break the heart. During these periods of uncertainty, the following may be noted.

- The skin on the balls of the feet can become rubbery due to:
  - not feeling oneself
  - putting on a pretence that everything is fine even though deep down it doesn't feel that way.
- Sores reveal fresh hurts whether on the body or the feet.
- Scars are reminders of old war wounds that linger because, at some level, there is a reluctance to heal.
- Ulceration indicates that certain emotions are still gnawing away on the inside.
- Swellings, lumps and bumps highlight areas of emotional congestion.
- Dirt on the balls of the feet:
  - covers up vulnerability
  - hides self-consciousness
  - shows areas of disgust.

- Bits of grass that cling to the balls of the feet indicate unnecessary emotions that can be easily discarded.
- Temporary markings, usually from socks or shoes, are fleeting impressions or reminders; for instance:
  - the weave of the sock can leave the momentary impression of being emotionally caught up
  - a line from the stocking could indicate a transitory division.
- Oedematous balls of the feet come from a buildup of fluid that can make these parts look really heavy, especially when overwhelmed by unresolved emotions.

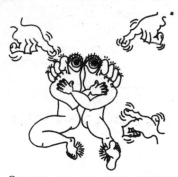

CRITICISM CAN BE SO SOUL DESTROYING.

MORE SENSITIVE ISSUES

The skin is likely to harden when going through a hard time or having to deal with ongoing hardships; whereas rough patches roughen the skin when it is too difficult to deal with an emotionally fraught situation or when there is excessive strain or awkwardness.

- Hard skin develops on the balls of the feet:
  - to fiercely protect identity or time and space, especially on those who care and look after others
  - to show the difficulty in catching one's breath
  - when being so caught up in the material world results in heartlessness.
- Calluses are emotional barriers against callous behaviour.
- Isolated patches of hard skin highlight highly-sensitive areas related to some specific emotive issue.

The inner conflict of mixed emotions when putting on a brave front
and pretending that nothing is wrong can cause the skin to keep
thickening and become extremely hard, often giving the impression of
being unfeeling, thick-skinned, hard-hearted, impenetrable, defensive
or even stubborn; yet deep down there is a tremendous amount of
hurt. Soft, pliable skin, at the other extreme, helps adapt more
spontaneously; being too soft, however:

- could mean that others take advantage
- may indicate a lack of substance
- is possibly due to a fear of standing one's ground
- is from having to tread carefully to survive.

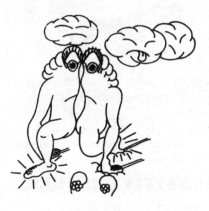

WEIGHED DOWN BY HEFTY EMOTIONS.

TIP

It is best to deal with the remnants of the past now, first by
thanking oneself and then by appreciating those who have created
the awareness of the inner shame, hurt, abandonment and so on.

LEAVING A MARK

Certain events and experiences make a profound impression, leaving their mark on the mind, body and soul, which is then reflected onto the soles. This is where they will stay until something is done about the situation. Should they have a detrimental effect then they can hinder progress and need to be sorted out before causing damage.

- Lines on the balls of the feet indicate:
  - concern, worry or anxiety
  - an emotional division or separation
  - where a line is drawn emotionally
  - areas that are fraught with tension
  - secretive parts of oneself
  - deeply-contained feelings.
- Horizontal lines are a sign of:
  - emotional ties
  - extreme anxiety
  - a need to feel the way step by step
  - emotional confusion
  - keeping the lid on mixed feelings in order to cope.
- Deep fissures or distinct vertical lines on the balls of the feet indicate intense emotion from:
  - feeling cut up and divided
  - being pulled apart after a divorce, death, separation, moving countries or some other major change
  - leading a double life and living in two very different environments.
- Vertical lines that extend into the insteps reveal that emotions are interfering and getting in the way of whatever's going on.
- Random lines usually indicate emotional confusion, with a whirlwind and volcanic effect.
- Crossed lines could be from being at:
  - cross-purposes
  - crossroads
  - feeling cross.
- A crucifix is a probable cross to bear, such as an elderly parent, a disadvantaged child, an alcoholic spouse and so on.

- A circle may suggest:
  - emotionally going around in circles
  - working around a particularly sensitive issue
  - the completion of something touchy.
- Stars are likely to indicate:
  - star-crossed love
  - well-blessed circumstances.

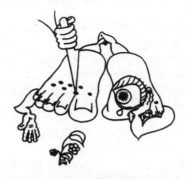

LINES AND MARKS REVEAL SOMETHING SO MUCH DEEPER.

NOTE

As the soul leaves the body at death, all the impressions and tensions of the physical world usually dissipate, leaving the soles smooth, colourless and unblemished, unless the soul is moving on to a completely different dimension, in which case, all the impressions remain on the feet.

A FEEL FOR THE THYMUS GLAND REFLEXES

The thymus gland is considered to be the seat of the soul since it radiates the true essence. It is also believed to be the centre of love that spreads passion throughout the whole body for greater appreciation of oneself and others. This automatically boosts feelings of self-worth and favourably affects the stature of the body and feet.

The reflexes for the thymus gland are midway down the central portion of both feet, where a slight hollow can be felt, unless feeling vulnerable, in which case it will be more solid or have hard skin. Issues only arise when feeling under attack for not being good enough, whilst bunions displace these reflexes so much that the soul really feels out of place.

- Hard skin forms over the thymus gland reflexes when protecting oneself.
- A thumbprint over these reflexes indicates that somebody is trying to superimpose their own identity.
- These reflexes swell when subconsciously reaching out for assistance, attention or sympathy.
- They sink when feeling that the soul is destroyed.

Appreciation and love is the best way to boost self-esteem and self-worth, bringing out the very best in individuals.

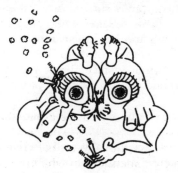

NOT BEING TRUE TO ONESELF.

NOTE

Concentrate on massaging these reflexes whilst visualizing pure green. For those with aids, ME or lupus this may help boost their immune system and feel better in themselves.

TAKING IN LIFE FORCE ENERGIES

Breathing and eating are expressions of life that symbolize the taking in of new experiences, which are essential for personal growth and development. Air boosts the morale whilst food provides the inner strength and resourcefulness to get through life's challenges and rediscover the spirit. The reflexes for the airways and oesophagus extend from the bases of the big toes to the fleshy insteps, along the inside edges of both balls of the feet, revealing the impact of innermost emotions that, if too overwhelming, can make one choke.

- The oesophageal and airway reflexes swell when emotionally overwhelmed.
- They sink, look pale or even white, when:
  - tired of having to take in the same old thing
  - swallowing a lot of nonsense
  - unsavoury things are constantly shoved down the throat.
- Hard skin develops over these reflexes when emotionally fraught, making it difficult to breath and hard to swallow.
- A ridge of skin acts as a cover-up for deep hurt.
- A bunion displaces the thymus gland reflexes and indicates:
  - going the long way round or in a roundabout way to express one's true feelings
  - subconsciously trying to break free, having had an extremely restrictive upbringing
  - a highly principled and exceptionally well-disciplined soul
  - extreme prejudice, intense intolerance or exceptional bias
  - feeling emotionally trapped within oneself.

When aligned with one's divine self it makes it so much easier to show respect to oneself and others.

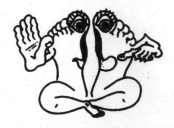

PREVENTED FROM TAKING IN THE FULLNESS OF LIFE.

THE BREATH OF LIFE

Without the breath, it is impossible to exist. Yet, it's the way in which the breath is taken in that determines the quality of life, since breathing is intricately linked to feelings about oneself and others. This is why emotions can be a matter of life and death. They influence the rhythm of the breath, determine the distribution of air throughout the whole body, and affect the heartbeat, as well as blood pressure and circulation, whilst also impinging on digestion. Ripples of emotion constantly spread throughout the body conveying innermost feelings to all the cells, although some are kept close to the chest, which then fill the air whenever breathing out. These emotions give a feel for the surrounding environment and, by connecting to the outer world, allow the inner world to be explored for greater familiarity with the stranger aspects of oneself. The buoyancy of the lung reflexes, on the balls of the feet, reveal how good one feels about oneself and others.

- Rigid, unbending lung reflexes are often a pain to walk on because of:
  – extreme emotional insecurity
  – a lack of self-worth.
- Emotional congestion makes these reflexes appear heavy and engorged due to:
  – keeping a host of unaired emotions to oneself
  – the strain of being there for so many people.
- Swollen lung reflexes is a sign of needing more space; with the heaviness often dragging the balls of the feet down, until the upper parts of the feet are no longer visible.
- The lung reflexes bulge when desperately reaching out for more love and attention.
- These parts look drained, flat and deflated when:
  – completely sapped of energy
  – weary and exhausted from constantly being at the beck and call of others
  – tried of having to keep a tight grip on one's feelings.

Certain breathing techniques, along with reflexology, relax the mind, body and soul, ridding them of toxic emotions and creating the space to reconnect with innermost feelings, as well as the essence of the spirit.

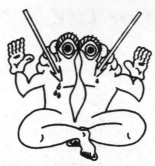

BEING STABBED IN THE CHEST MAKES IT DIFFICULT TO BREATHE!

MIRRORED ONTO THE BREAST REFLEXES

Breasts, whether male or female, contain the most profound and deepest affections, with their size and shape being linked to the emotional environment. Sharing the same reflexes as the lungs, they too occupy the bulk of the central mounds on both balls of the feet, revealing the amount of appreciation for oneself and others. They rely greatly on loving energies, with their appearance showing a balance between caring for loved ones and taking care of one's own innermost needs. This is where poor self-esteem can get in the way, even in the most loving of environments.

- Hard skin develops over the nipple reflexes, in the centres of the balls of the feet, to subconsciously:
  - stop others from taking advantage
  - avoid being sucked dry
  - put a stop to being sucked in.
- The balls of the feet wrinkle with:
  - concern about other people's feelings
  - extreme emotional anxiety that drains one of vitality.

It is sometimes difficult to tell where the balls of the feet end and the insteps begin, especially when busily nurturing others, leaving no time or space to get on with one's own life, or when exceptionally passionate about everything. The breast reflexes are sometimes depicted on the tops of the feet, opposite the balls of the feet, which are the indirect or secondary reflexes that show where some of the more hurtful and devastating emotions have been shoved, along with a load of unshed tears and a great deal of heartfelt sadness.

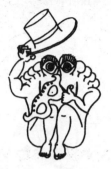

TAKING CARE OF ONESELF.

TROUBLED SOULS

Trouble starts when distressing emotions are kept close to the chest because they unnecessarily weigh down the mind, body and soul even though the problem invariably dates so far back that the details have long since been forgotten. However, with such an issue being made at the time, the affected tissue and cells remember until the memory is erased. However, horrific incidents are often kept alive through constantly being spoken about, with a danger of becoming so consumed with self-pity that the incident grows out of proportion and becomes quite sickening. When injured feelings entrap the soul then the role of victim is inevitable. Past hurts are continually used to torture the mind and hurt the body. If nothing is done about it then the uneasiness can get worse and develop into a full-blown disease.

Should the heftiness of these miserable feelings become really overwhelming, then the lower edges of the balls of the feet are likely to spread onto the insteps, to such an extent that the emotions get in the way of doing things; should it be the other way around, with the insteps impinging onto the balls of the feet, then the chances are that so much is being done for others that there is little or no room for oneself. Feelings have incredibly far-reaching effects, and either contaminate and pollute the atmosphere with gloomy, dreary or spiteful emotions that hang menacingly in the air, or clear the air with expressions of appreciation, love and joy, through the breath. Feet complain to draw attention to the fact that all is not well. Instead of going to a lot of trouble to please others, it is so much better to please oneself and the rest will follow.

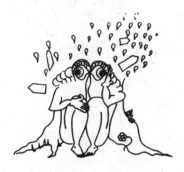

EMOTIONALLY DISTRAUGHT.

LOWER DOWN THE ARMS AND LEGS

The bottom halves of the lower arms and shins are deeply affected by feelings, even though the reflexes for both are in the communications and relationship parts of the feet. They reveal how feelings are relayed to others and rely on the flexibility of the wrists and ankles, as well as on the expansive movements of the shoulders and hips, to open up and make the most of every experience. Those things that are embraced and brought to the heart make it easier to breathe, whilst the emotionally-charged challenges that are kept at arm's length invariably cause inner turmoil. These parts of the body know when to reach out or hold back according to innermost feelings.

• The lower arm and leg reflexes protrude or swell when:
  – trying to keep things at a distance
  – tired of carrying hefty emotions.

Fortunately both the arms and legs are incredibly resourceful and powerful, they have the strength to reach out and help one stand up for oneself.

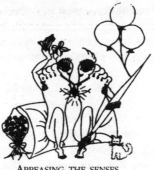

APPEASING THE SENSES.

TIP

Hugging holds to the heart those who are near and dear and, even when it's time to physically let go, the energy remains forever.

A LOOK AT THE UPPER BACK

The upper back reflexes extend over the tops of both feet, directly opposite the balls of the feet, to mirror emotional support and backing. It is here that the energy of unresolved emotions that are too painful or too horrendous to deal with reside. Hate, shame, guilt and fear, along with lost desires, are tucked back here causing a great deal of upper back discomfort and problems.

- These upper back reflexes are painful or ache when:
  - feeling emotionally stabbed in the back
  - the back has been turned on somebody important or significant
  - shoving a whole load of unresolved issues behind one's back.
- They collapse when:
  - overwhelmed with emotion
  - feeling a lack of emotional support
  - giving in under the strain of too much emotional responsibility.
- Black marks or freckles:
  - are a sign of deep hurt from a previous life experience

- highlight areas of weakness, which, once dealt with, puts one
  in a much stronger position; for instance, a black mark on any
  of the communication reflexes could reveal a speech defect or
  difficulty in opening up; yet once overcome, the voice becomes
  one's fortune
- reveal disgrace, shame, dishonour, scandal, discredit, humiliation
  and disrepute.
- Unsightly veins on the tops of the feet reveal extreme sadness or
  nastiness that have been put in the background, yet keep popping
  up to show that they are now on their way out.
- Ligaments reveal one's belief in oneself, although they can look
  strained when used as iron rods for additional support during
  challenging times.
- Puffiness is due to unshed tears.
- Images and initials that show up on the upper back reflexes are
  connected to the energy of those loved ones who hover in the
  background, having moved on or passed over. They can show what
  is holding one back or reveal the support being offered.

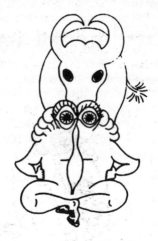

THE UNIVERSE PROVIDES ONGOING SUPPORT AND BACKING.

FEELING SO MUCH BETTER

Too often the greatest pain to overcome is the pain of disliking oneself, which is invariably portrayed through certain dislikes in others. If this doesn't make sense, then look to the shadow side, which hovers illusively in the background, until attention is drawn to it by what is thought, said or done. It is impossible to recognize characteristics in others unless they are a part of oneself, just as it's hard to understand a foreign language unless acquainted with it. It is through mirroring that individuals get to know themselves better since everybody has a good and bad side. If one keeps looking for what's wrong in others, they will find it; whereas, looking for the good in them means it's more likely to bring out the best in them.

From time to time hurt feelings do come to the fore, not to be dwelt upon and magnified, but to be understood and learnt from, so that they can be released with love. Feet are such a help at times like this because they show what's wrong and provide the insight to heal old wounds. The more one accepts oneself and others, the more it enhances the healing. Loving feelings nourish the emotional body, increase inner strength and boost immunity, which uplifts the spirits, brightens the eyes, improves circulation and helps digestion, all of which promotes inner harmony. Feeling better about oneself makes it so much easier to believe and trust in others.

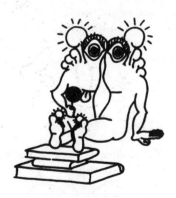

BEING ONESELF FEELS GREAT!

07 Deep in the heart – the bridge between the body and the spirit

AT THE HEART OF IT ALL

The heart reflexes are soft palpable mounds, about the size of a fingertip, situated where the balls of the feet meet the insteps. The left reflex is more prominent since the heart is mainly on the left side of the body. The heart is referred to as the spirit's mind, since the content or discontent of the mind affects the overall characteristics of the heart and affects its ability to perform.

These reflexes are energetically linked to:

• the second toes and fingers along with the balls of the feet
• the third toes and fingers, as well as the upper halves of the insteps.

The heart is a very sentimental part of the body that functions according to memories and the feelings that come with them. Fortunately the ever-accommodating heart is able to refine these emotions since it acts as the transformer of the body. Furthermore, being almost in the centre of the body, it is well aware of everything that is going on in the mind and the rest of the body, with blood acting as its messenger. In this way the heart can keep beating and provide the impetus to live life to the full.

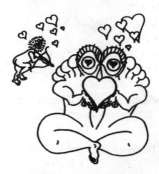

WITH ALL ONE'S HEART.

THE HEAD VERSUS THE HEART

A dreadful or fearful state of mind adversely affects the heart, making it sore, especially when there is conflict between the two. Even though the heart thrives on love and gratitude, the head is not always prepared to give it. Also the mind tends to dwell in the past or zoom into the future, yet the heart functions at its best in the present. Angry, revengeful and disturbing notions constrict the heart, often giving the impression of being uncaring and hard-hearted.

As the blood rushes to the face when embarrassed and as the body gets uptight, the cells begin to panic, as their supply of essential life forces rapidly diminishes, which further distresses the heart. Any form of emotional hurt or abuse makes this situation worse, often leading to the belief that life is traumatic and filled with nothing but ongoing distress. The heart takes a great deal of strain when sickness becomes the focal point of concern and finds it extremely difficult to cope.

- Swollen heart reflexes reveal:
  - a mass of unresolved emotions getting in the way
  - heartache due to built-up resentment
  - difficulty in overcoming heart-rending situations that pull at the heartstrings.
- Hard skin develops over these reflexes:
  - as a means of protection
  - to prevent hard-heartedness.
- A deep crevice or cut, just beneath the heart reflexes, reveals devastation or being emotionally cut up when cut off because of a divorce, death or separation.
- More than one cut is a sign of:
  - feeling emotionally cut off
  - not wishing to get involved with ongoing drama
  - attempting to sever emotions to cope with a fraught emotional environment.
- A line may appear through these reflexes to reveal a broken heart.
- Tiny blood vessels or miniscule 'droplets of blood' are a sign of a bleeding heart.
- Hardened reflexes indicate a hardening of the heart in an attempt to survive or subconsciously prevent any further heartache.

This can all change in a heartbeat, by filling the mind with appreciative, kind thoughts that relax the whole body and make it kindhearted.

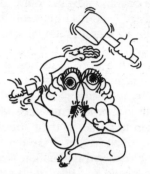

THINKING WITH THE HEAD OR THE HEART MAKES A BIG DIFFERENCE.

THE TEMPERAMENT AT HEART

Depending on the heart's temperament, feet can either be warm or boiling hot one moment and freezing cold the next, according to how easily riled or placid one is. Everybody is capable of both extremes. Heat fires the heart and gets things going, yet too much, generated through anger, fury or extreme passion, can make the blood boil. Heat causes the feet to burn with passion and desire or an all-consuming need for revenge. Coolness, meanwhile, dampens the spirit and slows the heart, especially when depressed, unhappy or miserable, whereas doom and gloom depress the heart and dull the spirit.

- Hot feet often turn bright red showing that:
  - intense feelings are getting the better of one
  - there is suppression of deep fury, frustration or resentment.
- Cold feet indicate a short supply of get up and go, with many worthwhile projects being aborted, due to:
  - deep unhappiness about being left out in the cold
  - extreme fear and anxiety
  - a complete lack of confidence
  - a reluctance to venture out on one's own
  - a lack of interest or enthusiasm
  - a dread at the thought of moving on.

- Blue feet are often a sign of cold feet but could also indicate deep emotional trauma and hurt, especially when accompanied by black marks.
- Feet can fluctuate from being icy cold to boiling hot whenever experiencing mixed emotions.
- Occasionally one foot may be hot and the other freezing cold, possibly from freezing at the thought of something that happened in the past, whilst becoming furious at the memory.

The heart loves it when the individual is animated, zealous and enthusiastic since these attributes really bring them to life.

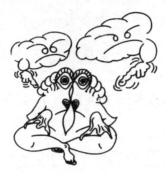

FILLING ONESELF WITH FEAR INSTEAD OF CONFIDENCE.

THE LOVE IN THE HEART

There is no getting away from it, wherever the body goes, the heart goes too. It constantly relays inner content or discontent to every cell, which is why, when filled with limitless love, then good health is inevitable. The moment there is any emotional pressure, the heart weakens and causes the whole body to suffer, affecting the characteristics of the feet.

The heart is the most important endocrine gland, with the atrial neuriatic factor influencing the entire hormonal system. This means that the more loving one is towards oneself and others, the more effective the heart becomes. Being totally honest with oneself about one's innermost feelings helps in getting through emotionally tumultuous times. Even though love itself doesn't hurt, it does allow one to feel the pain of not having love. So when relationships are good, circulation is good and there is an excellent flow of blood between the head and toes, which helps to clear the mind. Assisting the blood flow is the lymphatic system, the sewerage system of the body, that constantly removes anything detrimental to one's well-being, be it a toxic thought or a noxious emotion. Having a heart that never hardens, a temperament that is always consistent and a touch that never hurts is the best way to stay fit. Love, after all, is the most powerful force on earth and the greatest gift that one can give oneself and others.

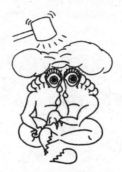

FIX A BROKEN HEART WITH LOVE.

DEEP WITHIN THE SOLAR PLEXUS

The solar plexus, known as the abdominal brain, is the hub of emotion that affects the nature of what is done or not done, as well as how it is done, all of which depends on whether one feels like it or not. Over an extended period of time, extreme emotions can upset the solar plexus and send it into an absolute tizz! Even though its true reflexes are immediately below the heart reflexes, the effect of emotions can be seen more clearly in the slight indentations immediately below the centres of the balls of the feet. These are the two most powerful reflexes in reflexology. Just placing a thumb or finger over these reflexes can effectively relax the entire being, mentally, emotionally, physically and spiritually, so much so that it can ease hyperventilation, an asthmatic attack or even a panic episode. Meanwhile the characteristics of these reflexes reveal how well the solar plexus is able to balance the emotions so that they don't interfere with the functioning of the digestive tract, especially during times of extreme concern or intense anxiety, since feelings such as these are likely to knot the stomach or cause butterflies.

There is also a fascinating symbolic connection between the solar plexus and the parable of the miraculous sharing of the five loaves and two fishes; with the five solar plexus ganglia nourishing the multitude of cells and two half moon ganglia bringing together the masculine and feminine sides of one's nature. The solar plexus is such a highly energetic part of the body that it can radiate tremendous energy throughout the whole, which contributes to a sunny disposition, as well as gut feel.

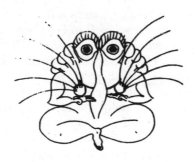

SUNSHINE AT THE VERY DEPTHS OF ONE'S BEING.

A PERPLEXED SOLAR PLEXUS

Discomfort around the solar plexus is often linked to the throat and the inability to speak up for oneself, along with self-centeredness, addictions, egocentricity, manipulation, lack of sleep, tension and phobias. These reflexes have much to 'say' when upset.

- The solar plexus reflexes swell when:
  - bogged down by the material aspects of life
  - hefty, unresolved emotions get in the way
  - unable to do what the soul desires.
- They sink when emotionally drained.
- Wavy lines over these reflexes indicate waves of emotion; feeling up in the air one moment and then down in the doldrums the next.
- Lines that extend downwards onto the upper insteps reveal:
  - emotional ties that get in the way of progress
  - the number of activities that are emotionally draining.

- Lines that stretch from the balls of the feet to the solar plexus reflexes represent the number of individuals who are emotionally dependent.
- Distinct lines or arcs over the tops of these reflexes occur when keeping somebody at bay.
- Dagger-shaped markings could be constant jabs and prods. When the dagger shape is reversed, the emotional digs could leave one breathless.
- Funnel-shaped lines that extend from the bases of the solar plexus reflexes are from having had the plug pulled and feeling flat and deflated.
- A line underneath the right solar plexus reflex, and another over the top of the left reflex, reveal the need to hold oneself up in the past but now having to protect oneself.
- Flaking skin over these reflexes reveals extreme irritation.
- The colour of the reflexes reveal emotions:
  - red solar plexus reflexes are a sign of extreme anger and frustration at feeling emotionally and physically out of control
  - these reflexes turn white when totally exhausted
  - bluish-purple reflexes reveal bruised emotions
  - yellow reflexes are from being exceptionally fed up at being manipulated
  - green solar plexus reflexes signify extreme envy that others are so much in control.

Once in control of oneself, physically, emotionally and spiritually, then the solar plexus reflexes should look firm, vibrant and well-balanced.

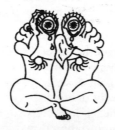

EMOTIONALLY OUT OF CONTROL.

COPING WITH HEARTFELT EMOTIONS

Emotions are thoughts that move through the body and stir memories as a reminder of how one felt in the past in similar situations. This fills the mind and body with hope, fear, dread or anticipation, to mention but a few of a wide range of emotions that then determine how the next step is taken. Everything is done from memory, be it a thought, feeling or action. It is memories that determine the quality of life. Frustration and disappointment, from expectations never being met, can cause a reluctance to get involved again, whilst really frightful memories can literally bring things to a standstill. The greatest fear is that of death, especially the death of the ego from dying of embarrassment.

Feeding the mind with past traumas is a measly diet for a healthy mind and body and starves the whole of vital sustenance. Past experiences are best used to gauge progress, so that one can become more of oneself. Beliefs can also play absolute havoc with the mind and body, even though a belief is only one point of view. Once there is no longer a need to always be 'right', a mutual respect can develop that does the heart and soul a world of good and is very reassuring for the solar plexus.

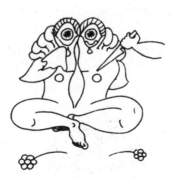

BELIEFS PLAY HAVOC WITH INNERMOST FEELINGS.

STEPS TO FEELING BETTER

Feeling vulnerable from time to time is a way of rediscovering one's own capabilities and regaining inner strength through resourcefulness. In this way there is greater understanding of the reason to be on earth. Pondering too much on the past or reflecting too often on the future immediately limits the present. Living in the moment expands time and makes it possible to achieve so much more; this, in turn, makes one feel so much better. It also brings to the fore quirky characteristics, plus the implementation of novel ideas, which are valid and feasible ways of gaining self-respect. Tension immediately dissipates, along with the ego and self-imposed limitations, allowing mind, body and soul to savour each breath. Once the individual fully embraces who and what they are, their heart becomes so full of love that they can't help but feel good!

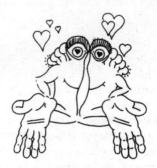

AT PEACE WITH ONESELF.

NOTE

The element of air is linked to the second fingers, which means that, when massaging feet, they can be used to calm and reassure, along with green, which soothes and creates space, and pink to infuse the whole with pure love. Also massaging the balls of the feet, to which the second toes and fingers are connected, eases inner emotional tension and boosts self-esteem. Meanwhile stroking the diaphragmatic reflexes provides more space in which to breathe. Finally, resting the thumbs or third fingers on the solar plexus reflexes helps to calm the whole being, especially whenever anxious or concerned.

08 The third toes – reflecting the liveliness of the mind

CONSTANTLY ON THE GO

The third toes reflect the idealistic, creative, social and romantic aspects of the mind, whilst their fiery qualities provide the passion and enthusiasm to get things done. This, in turn, fuels the mind and ensures sufficient energy to keep going. Being in the centres of both feet, these toes balance mind, body and spirit and immediately draw attention to anything that is not working in one's life. Their reputation as the 'doing' or 'active' toes links them to instinctive survival, as well as to self-actualization and self-realization. It takes a certain amount of determination, and a great deal of faith, to put extraordinary ideas to the test, but this is the only way to get to know oneself better. The third toes are energetically linked to the middle fingers, as well as the upper halves of the insteps and upper abdominal region.

They resonate to yellow, which is a particularly nurturing hue that brings out the sunny side of one's nature. The warmth of success helps the third toes stand flexibly upright, with their lengths showing the lengths they go to to make a difference. The longer the toes, the greater the potential for drive and energy. Meanwhile the more rounded the third toe pads the more well rounded the individual. Being an ongoing success brings out the best. These toes help think things through and serve as an excellent reminder of innermost capabilities.

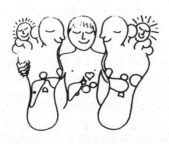

FULL OF AMBITION.

TRIALS OF BEING THIRD

It is so much easier to keep going and make the most of life when feeling good about oneself and others. The moment there is any doubt or a fear of not being good enough, then both the mind and body panic and become defensive, making it really difficult to get on and do what should be done. At times, although it's possible to get started, it can be impossible to keep going, because of not having the stamina or the interest. All of this is picked up by the third toes, which are forced to turn elsewhere or lean on the other toes for support. This could lead to frustration, resentment or retaliation, especially when prevented from doing things for oneself, which is why distorted third toes are fairly common on youngsters and the elderly.

• Third toes bend in shame, embarrassment or confusion when:
  – feeling inadequate
  – trying to please others for all the wrong reasons.
• Rigid third toes indicate:
  – inflexibility, stubbornness or single-mindedness
  – a perfectionist, who likes things done in a certain way
  – insecurity or selfishness, set ways that leave no room for other people's ideas.
• These toes may appear battered when:
  – constantly critical
  – not believing in oneself and others down.
• They may look crooked due to:
  – things getting in the way
  – difficulty in getting the head around things
  – constantly having to twist and turn to adjust and adapt to unsuitable ways of thinking.
• Squashed third toes reveal:
  – being restricted when it comes to doing things
  – that the hands are tied
  – a fear of defying authority.
• Third toes look white and drained of colour and vitality when:
  – tired of being limited
  – exhausted from trying to convey unique notions.
• Yellow tinges are a sign of feeling really fed up.

- If these toes become hot and turn bright red it could be from:
  - extreme anger, frustration or embarrassment
  - hotheadedness and wanting to blow one's top.
- The third toes turn blue when:
  - feeling left out in the cold
  - experiencing cold feet.
- Bruised third toes indicate extreme hurt at not being taken seriously.

Blowing hot and cold can cause these toes to fluctuate between various colours and temperatures.

Some ladies have their middle toes amputated so that they can squeeze their feet into the latest pointed footwear, little realizing that this also cuts off their ability to think for themselves, yet to them outside validation is more important. Recognition, though, can only come from within, from feeling good about doing something worthwhile with one's life.

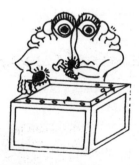

WHEN NO LONGER KNOCKING ONESELF, PROGRESS CAN BE MADE.

TIRED OF DOING SO MUCH

When it seems impossible to get ahead in life then look to the third toes to get an inkling of why this is.

- Third toes knock the second toes when berating oneself or taking it out on others.
- The second toes knock the third toes showing that one may feel incompetent and not believe in oneself.

- Third toes overlap the second toes, showing that a brave front is being put on in order to get things done.
- Third toes overshadow the second toes when the ego or feelings of inadequacy restrict activities.
- Third toes support the second toes when self-esteem needs bolstering.
- Third toes bump the fourth toes due to:
  - constant criticism and censorship
  - being bumped off a project
  - an attempt to retaliate.
- Fourth toes hammer the third toes when bullied into doing things against one's will.
- Third toes overlap the fourth toes when:
  - keeping mum about something charitable or completely unacceptable
  - work takes a precedence over relationships.
- Fourth toes overshadow the third toes revealing:
  - extreme shyness or self-consciousness
  - a lot of talk but little or no action.
- Third toes stand back, when:
  - holding back
  - extremely uncertain
  - concerned about other people's opinions
  - fearful of being disgraced or rejected.
- These toes stand alone:
  - in a display of individuality
  - due to feeling lonely or abandoned.
- Hard skin appears on the tips of the third toes:
  - concealing the agitation of not being able to think for oneself
  - preventing ideas from being knocked.
- Corns form on the tops of these toes:
  - to stop others from treading on the toes and, therefore, personal notions
  - when independent ways of thinking are being stamped out.

For two people to think alike and completely understand one another is an impossibility, although they can be on the same wavelength and contribute unique ideas when it comes to doing things, providing the ideal basis for expansion.

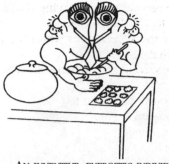

AN INVENTIVE, ENERGETIC INDIVIDUAL.

IN STEP WITH THE SOUL'S DESIRES

The naturally vibrant and lively third toes are energetically connected to the upper halves of the insteps, which reveal the affects of one's actions and reactions, and whether these are empowering or disempowering them. If life has become a bore the chances are that the soles are worn out from doing the same old thing day in and day out, instead of having the gumption to explore new ground and be different. The subconscious part of the mind constantly wanders to the emotional parts of the body (reflected onto the second toes and balls of the feet) and then refers to the communicative parts (mirrored on the fourth toes and lower halves of the insteps) to determine one's feelings about doing something before a decision is made. The constant to-ing and fro-ing of the mind means that every situation can be fully assessed, based on what went on in the past, enabling the third toes to provide a balance no matter what happens. This is so much easier when in one's element and doing what one loves, which allows the upper digestive track to function as it should. The primary reflexes for the alimentary canal are on the upper halves of the sole insteps, whilst the secondary reflexes are immediately opposite these on the tops of the feet. The former reveal the capacity of dealing with everyday activities, whilst the latter draw attention to anything untoward that is going on in the background, as well as the amount of backup when it comes to doing things. The right upper instep discloses the influence of past events on current behaviour, whilst the left upper instep shows what's going on now.

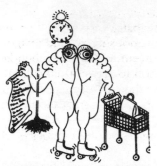

MAKING THE MOST OF EVERYTHING.

AFFECTING THE UPPER HALVES OF THE INSTEPS

Not being able to make the mind up and being indecisive is very unsettling, whilst the impact of all that is done or not done affects the vibrancy, appearance and pliability of the upper halves of the insteps, especially on the soles.

- The upper halves of the insteps wrinkle with concern or worry.
- A deep vertical division appears when:
  - having no idea of which way to turn
  - pulled in two completely different directions
  - there is a conflict of interests.
- Lines are usually a sign of:
  - being cut up and divided
  - drawing the line when it comes to doing things
  - feeling tied down
  - being involved in various projects that are worlds apart or have nothing to do with one another.
- Lines that extend:
  - from the outer edges indicate commitments, concerns or ties regarding the family or society
  - from the inner edges are more intellectually orientated.
- A horizontal line, stretching across the upper halves of the insteps, appears when:
  - feeling stretched

– cut in half
– not wishing to participate.
- To find out what the various marks and images mean, ask the individual what they mean to them and then keep questioning.
- Swellings draw attention to areas of difficulty because of things getting in the way or when life seems like an up-hill slog:
  – the size of the bump gives an indication of the enormity of what's going on
  – the number of bumps show the number of obstacles that get in the way
  – the position of the bulges reveals whether the challenge is intellectual (if under the big toes), emotional (if under the second toes) and so on.
- A thorn in this area could mean:
  – a thorn in the side
  – feeling under attack for not being good enough.
- A splinter may be from:
  – feeling fragmented
  – a chip on one's shoulder
  – resentment at being a chip off the old block.
- These areas become red when:
  – fuming about what's going on or about something that happened in the past
  – burning with infuriation
  – suppressed anger gets in the way.
- Cramping stems from extreme fear:
  – of others cramping one's style
  – of not being able to perform as well as expected.

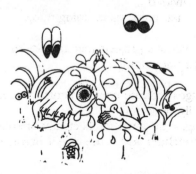

LOST SOULS WITH LITTLE OR NO SENSE OF DIRECTION.

AS FEET TAKE SHAPE

The shape of the feet depends on the shape that the individual is in, according to what is going on in their mind, as well as their type of personality. As things take shape, their feet use some or all of their 26 small bones, 19 muscles and 30 plus ligaments, to adapt themselves and fit into the ever-changing needs, whilst also providing a balanced surface and firm platform from which anything and everything can be handled. The only thing that gets in their way is a negative state of mind, which alters the outline of the feet to such an extent that it can be too difficult or painful to stand. Other factors that influence the shape of the feet are upbringing and cultural beliefs, along with inherent attitudes, and the impact of past events. A flexible mind relaxes the feet allowing them to remain versatile, supple and complaisant. If, however, they are too flexible, there is a risk of being too malleable and easily manipulated. Rigidity, meanwhile, indicates uncertainty, extreme insecurity, a strict upbringing or a highly-principled individual. The stiffer the feet, the less they can bend and the more troublesome they become, which tends to make it difficult to progress.

When feet are supple, they are more capable of withstanding the knocks of life. It is only when things get to be too much that the feet take on the contortions of the mind, along with the agony of forcing oneself to conform and fit in to conflicting, unsuitable belief systems that stem from harsh ethnic, social or parental notions. Swellings are a way of trying to get on top of unpleasant situations, whilst shrivelling is a sign of giving in to constant constraints and restrictions. Either way, the shape and appearance of the feet can change quite dramatically. Meanwhile, the condition of the feet reflect whether the soul is in good shape because, as actions take shape, the feet adjust to accommodate the vast range of movements. Since everybody has their own way of doing things, each pair of feet is unique, but overall it is possible to see the shape of things to come by looking at the overall shape of feet.

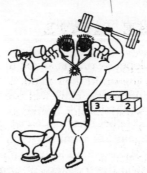

STAYING IN SHAPE.

OUTLINING THE VARIOUS SHAPES

Well-proportioned feet easily assimilate abstract knowledge and provide a firm foundation on which to move. As they constantly change their appearance they are able to keep pace with ongoing needs, with their outline revealing the current frame of mind.

• Broad, supple feet indicate:
  – a broad-minded, down-to-earth soul
  – a capacity to deal with almost anything
  – being grounded enough to act spontaneously
  – a broad basis from which to function
  – a soul who likes to assist others, especially those who are less fortunate
  – a hard worker with good organizational skills
  – somebody who prefers not to get too involved if hectically busy.
• Overly broad feet tend to:
  – overcompensate in order to survive
  – believe that a great impression needs to be made
  – make sure that everything is well covered.
• Narrow feet show:
  – a more sensitive and gentle soul, with an aesthetic appreciation of life
  – a love of being pampered
  – the tendency to narrow things down to find a delicate balance
  – an inclination to tread carefully
  – an ability to move quickly to get out of harm's way

- limited space in which to function
- self-imposed restraints and restrictions
- precise and exact ways of doing things
- a great deal of attention to detail.

Traditionally some Chinese women had their feet cruelly bound because they were considered to be subservient and were bound by tradition and strict social belief systems at that time. Their miniscule feet show just how insignificant women were in the greater scheme of things. Today ballet dancers tend to have misshapen feet as they desperately try to follow in the footsteps of prima ballerinas, although this aptly mirrors their set ideas and pedantic ways. It helps to take into account culture, upbringing and belief systems when assessing the shape of feet, since they all provide a general outline and show where the individual is coming from.

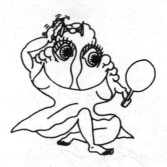

THE MIND SHAPES THE FUTURE AND THE FEET.

OTHER PARAMETERS TO CONSIDER

There are so many different shapes to take into account that it is far better to be intuitively guided and see what comes to mind.

- Functional feet, with large soles but insignificant-looking toes, do so much for others that there is little or no time to think for themselves.
- Philosophical feet, with large, distinctive toes, have insignificant-looking soles revealing:
  - great ideas but difficulty in doing anything worthwhile with them

  – amazing concepts that are so unusual that they are generally kept
    to oneself.
- Psychic feet with flat-topped toes and long necks that give them a
  funnel-shaped appearance, that are invariably linked to the spiritual
  realms of consciousness.
- Straight and narrow feet indicate:
  – a more straightforward, no-nonsense approach to life
  – the need to set parameters and stay within the straight and narrow
  – a direct approach to life
  – the tendency to take umbrage to anything that is not on the
    agenda.

(Track runners often have this type of feet.) Most feet are a mixture of
shapes. For instance, they could have philosophical toes with short,
practical necks but their soles could be unusually elegant because,
although they have the ability to escape in their mind, they also have
a very practical and down-to-earth approach allowing them to use
their amazing ideas in the most charming and intricate ways.

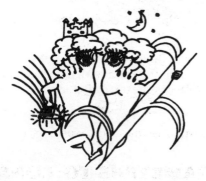

PSYCHIC AND INTUITIVE FEET, WITH THEIR HEADS IN THE CLOUDS.

OUT OF SHAPE

Trying to conform and squeeze into unsuitable belief systems does
neither the individual nor their feet any good. However this happens
so frequently that there are many lost souls wandering aimlessly
around, who have been sorely misguided, fearfully conditioned or
inexcusably downtrodden. The more misshapen the feet, the more
unhappy and disillusioned the individual tends to be, with the

weightiness of everything becoming too much that it eventually becomes impossible to take another step.

• Feet become misshapen when under pressure due to:
  – the mind trying to adapt into other ways of thinking
  – a desperate attempt to fit in, even though this is ultimately impossible
  – feeling unworthy, rejected, deprived or abandoned, as well as out of place
  – going though a rough patch
  – having a relentless grip on things
  – testing oneself to see how far one can go without getting hurt.
• Feet that have been deformed since birth indicate that during the pregnancy the mother may have:
  – had some unbearable restraints and restrictions imposed on her
  – gone through a terrifying time
  – felt completely helpless in the circumstances she found herself in.
• Numbness in the feet comes from cutting oneself off from feeling the pain of the past.
• Paralysis stems from a profound fear that literally stops one in their tracks.

The shape and state of the body and feet are influenced by memories and beliefs that the feet help to put into perspective so that the mind and body can move on to the next stage of life.

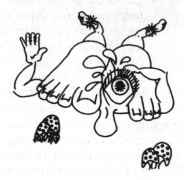

TIRED AND EXHAUSTED FROM TRYING TO FIT IN.

> **NOTE**
>
> Massaging the feet daily, with cream, encourages them to gradually change shape as the soothing movements ease the mind, relax the body and reassure the soul, until there is no longer a need to conform to out-dated and unreasonable beliefs, leaving the soles, and the soul, free to shape their own future.

ASSESSING THE LIVER REFLEXES

The liver is an extremely sentimental part of the body, containing remnants of the past, along with a hoard of amassed tales that have been passed on by family and friends. It brims with energy that comes from prior accomplishments and successes, which it uses to recharge the mind, body and soul. With the liver being so full of what happened or didn't happen in the past, it resides mainly on the right side of the body, consistently processing the consequences of every event, as well as the effects of any non-event. Its slightly domed, triangular-shaped reflex shows up mainly on the right foot, filling the outer half and inner upper quadrant of that instep; with a much smaller triangular-shaped portion overlapping a part of the stomach reflex, on the left foot.

The insight that can be gained as to why certain events took place, whilst others didn't, helps to balance one's appetite for life. It's the past that fuels the present, providing the drive and enthusiasm to keep going in an attempt to get better at being oneself. However, from time to time, less pleasant memories can get in the way and, in the process of being worked out, may stir some deep-seated primitive responses, such as anger, frustration and resentment. These immediately change the tempo of what is going on, which inevitably affects the type of energy generated in the liver and simultaneously changes the characteristics of the reflexes. Hanging onto past experiences for fear of losing one's identity or designated role in life, be it a self-professed victim or self-assured victor, saps the body of energy, causing the liver reflexes to sink. It is then virtually impossible to extract any form of heat or enthusiasm from the liver, which can then lead to ongoing tiredness and utter exhaustion. It's the attitude that either revs or switches off mind, body and soul and determines the amount of 'liveliness' as one 'livens up' and comes to life.

✱ 139

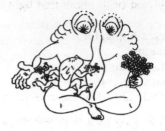

A LIVELY EXISTENCE!

LACKING ENERGY

It can be extremely discouraging to eat the freshest and most
wholesome of foods yet still have no energy; whilst eating nothing at
all can really energize the body. This is because it's the passion that
comes from doing things that ultimately enthuses and energizes the
whole being. The livelier one is, the more effective the liver. Constant
resentment makes the liver highly volatile and increasingly prone to
outbursts of anger, some of which can be accompanied by screaming
fits. Depression may then follow due to being in the dark as to why
certain things are happening and others aren't.

- The right liver reflex swells when:
  - there's difficulty in working things through the system because of
    refusing to let go of the past
  - unable to sort things out in the mind
  - detoxifying or on a strict vegan diet.
- The main liver reflex sinks from:
  - being tired, drained and exhausted from taking on too much
  - doing the same old thing time and time again.
- These reflexes turn yellow because of:
  - a jaundiced outlook
  - feeling really fed up
  - the situation has become bad enough to drive one to drink
  - self-rejection that can lead to an addictive personality and the
    misuse of substances.
- The liver reflex becomes bright red when fuming at having to do
  things that go against the grain or when highly energized.

- This reflex may turn orange when extremely annoyed with all that what went on in the past or to show that light has been thrown on a situation.
- Hardened liver reflexes highlight:
  – impenetrable emotions
  – tough situations that make one cynical
  – an attitude of 'what's the use, anyway?'
  – the difficulty of getting ahead because of what went on in the past.

Looking back is okay, as long as it is to see the amount of progress made and to realize just how much has been achieved.

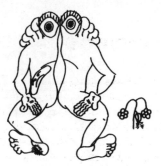

NOBODY CARES.

CONSIDER THE GALL BLADDER REFLEX

The liver processes everything that is going on inside the body so that it can derive as much information as possible to keep things going. It even has the gall to examine and debrief the red blood cells to find out how happy the mind, body and soul are about everything that has taken place. The results of this interrogation is bile, which is temporarily stored in a tiny sac, known as the gall bladder, embedded in the centre of the liver, before it moves into the duodenum, where it acts as the 'ambassador' of the body. It's by drawing on past experiences that the incoming food knows what to expect, which then determines the reaction, as well as the chemical make-up and composition of the body, according to the amount of satisfaction and fulfilment derived. Resentment has a bitterness that creates a very putrid environment, in which things rot easily, causing extreme dissatisfaction.

Although the gall bladder reflex is barely visible, it can be felt as a miniscule palpable ball midway along an imaginary line that extends diagonally across the right instep. This reflex hardens or become highly sensitive when there is an unusually large amount of bitterness about what was previously done or not done, or accumulated indignation about some really offensive behaviour. This can be prevented by making the most of every opportunity, which helps in dealing with the unexpected.

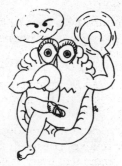

FULL OF ANGER AND RESENTMENT.

STOMACHING LIFE

The stomach provides instant energy when it comes to dealing with everyday circumstances, as well as with anything that is taken on board. It provides firsthand knowledge of all the options available as it first sorts things out, processes them and finally integrates them. All this happens according to innermost feelings and the manner in which these are relayed, which then affects the way in which experiences are stomached and deciphered. The body relies on the fiery qualities of the stomach to provide an intense desire to get the very best out of life, which then fuels mind, body and soul and ensures that there is more than enough energy and enthusiasm to keep going.

The stomach is appropriately situated on the present side of the body, with its reflexes being mainly on the left foot, showing how well it accepts or rejects whatever comes its way. A tiny part of the stomach reflex then extends across to the corresponding area on the right instep, to reveal how the leftovers of the past influence the current situation. Meanwhile the cardiac sphincter reflexes, at the junction between the balls of the feet and insteps, guard the entrance of the stomach, whilst those for the pyloric sphincter, at the base of the right ball of the foot, in line with the junction of the second and big toes, help to keep things moving.

- The cardiac sphincter reflexes swell when:
  - overwhelmed by the enormity of all that is having to be stomached
  - feeling out of control
  - suffering from heartburn because of a burning issue that strains the heart and causes a reflux of bitterness that makes the oesophagus too acidic.
- If one is emotionally severed or pulled apart this may cause a hiatus hernia. In this case the pyloric sphincter reflexes swell:
  - when unable to process what's going on
  - feeling ill prepared
  - not being too happy about moving onto the next stage.
- The cardiac sphincter reflexes collapse when:
  - so busy caring for others that there is no time for oneself
  - tired of the monotony of having to do the same old thing time and time again.
- The pyloric sphincter gives in because of
  - not having the strength to keep things moving
  - a kick in the stomach.

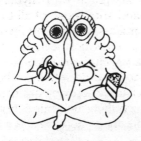

TAKING IT ALL IN.

IN THE PIT OF THE STOMACH

Anxiety arises from a fear of not being able to cope, especially when there is nervousness about a forthcoming event, such as going to a new school, writing an exam, starting another job, getting married, moving home or having a baby, any of which can upset the tummy. Furthermore, feeling out of control makes it seem far more difficult to cope, especially when there is a backlog of things to do, all of which amount to bloatedness or extra padding around the girth as a form of protection.

- The main stomach reflex swells when:
  - overwhelmed at having to stomach so much
  - there is too much on one's plate
  - having no idea which way to turn
  - having had a gut full
  - unable to deal with unresolved issues concerning one's mother.
- This same reflex collapses when:
  - drained at the thought of all that has gone on
  - feeling kicked in the stomach
  - utterly exhausted from doing so much for others
  - things eat away at one with the possibility of a gastric ulcer.
- Lines across the stomach reflexes usually indicate:
  - the number of activities that have been taken on
  - the manner in which jobs are divided so that they can be done one by one
  - being pulled in many directions
  - feeling really caught up in what is being done, especially if the lines look like a net.
- Hardened stomach reflexes are a sign of extreme difficulty because of feeling so tied down.
- Wrinkles of concern cover this reflex when exceptionally anxious about what is going on.
- A deep crevice between the stomach and heart reflexes could be a way of:
  - preventing any further heartbreak
  - not allowing emotions to get in the way of what needs to be done
  - avoiding emotional involvement with what is going on, which is why it is commonly found on medical personnel who handle many heartbreaking situations as part of their daily duties.

- Faint, random lines could be flutters of uneasiness about having to deal with certain things.
- Colours indicate the underlying emotion:
  - red stomach reflexes reveal extreme anger and frustration at what's going on or exceptional energy
  - the stomach reflexes look white when tired, drained and exhausted or to show divine intervention
  - whitish-yellow pockets are signs of accumulated resentment
  - blue stomach reflexes show the hurt at being criticized and judged
  - yellow tinges appear on these reflexes when totally fed up or to show enlightenment.

If the stomach has a problem, the whole body is affected since it is the hub of everything that happens, which is why it so willingly fortifies each atom of the body from top to toe.

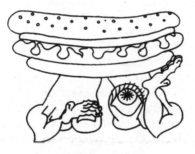

MORE THAN A GUT FULL!

COURAGE FROM THE ADRENAL GLANDS

The adrenal glands provide the guts with a sense of belief and innovation despite the trepidation that may be felt inside. Even though they have long out-grown the 'flight or fight' reputation, inner turmoil can still remain, along with the fear of failure. However, these glands are the first to provide the courage and superhuman strength to put extraordinary ideas into action, no matter what!

Their reflexes are perched on top of the kidney reflexes (page 23), just beneath the solar plexus reflexes, with the right adrenal reflex being fractionally lower and slightly nearer the inner edge of the foot than that of the left adrenal reflex.

- The adrenal gland reflexes enlarge or swell when:
  - fear gets in the way
  - trying to overcompensate
  - needing to be extra resourceful
  - in a particularly demanding situation
  - constantly having to protect oneself
  - there are incessant arguments
  - on guard against attack
  - trying to get through a crippling situation
  - blind and unable to see what's going on.
- These reflexes collapse and look drained on:
  - perfectionists who are never satisfied
  - those who continually compete even when there is no competition.

It is by becoming trustworthy that one becomes more trusting of others.

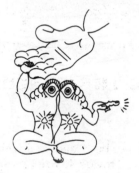

RECEIVING A HELPING HAND.

DUODENAL ANTICS

The duodenum acts as a vital link between the stomach and small intestines and, as such, connects the essence of all that is done to the way in which current relationships are nurtured. The actual C-shape of this reflex follows the outline of the inner, upper quadrant of the right instep and, although it is not generally visible, it is an area that can ache when longing for something different to happen yet not having the courage to do anything about it. The duodenum is constantly aware of the impact of all that is done and uses this knowledge to make the most of the current circumstances, in the hope that there is no longer a need to slog away or begrudgingly work things through. Its length should provide enough time and space to get a grip on things and make the most of every situation. A duodenal ulcer may appear when the memories of the past become all consuming and gnaw away at the insides. This can be prevented from happening by giving appreciation for everything that happens, whilst also understanding why certain things don't happen.

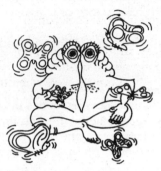

BUTTERFLIES IN THE STOMACH.

DELIGHTING THE PANCREATIC REFLEXES

The pancreas injects mind, body and soul with sweet thoughts that gratify the emotions and provide sufficient inspiration for the nectar of life to be absorbed. As such, it symbolizes the ability to attain the very best from each and every situation so that there is overall satisfaction and complete fulfilment. The contentment of this healthy situation soon becomes apparent on both the body and the feet, since it excites the heart and delights the muscles. The pancreatic reflexes are the slight mounds that are in the shape of a tadpole, which lie along the upper edges of both waistlines on the feet, with the broadest end in the centre of the right instep and tapering off to three-quarters of the way across the left instep.

They reveal the pancreas's ability to break down past experiences and show how it constantly strives to keep toxic thoughts and noxious emotions at bay so that they don't contaminate current experiences. The most persistent of these unhealthy notions come from hankering after the good old days, which are long since gone. So it is that the right pancreatic reflex mirrors the joy of all that was previously achieved, whilst the left pancreatic reflex reflects the amount of gratification received in the here and now. These reflexes are naturally vibrant and healthy looking, but are easily upset by emotionally-fraught circumstances or traumatic experiences.

• The pancreatic reflexes distend when attempting to:
  – reach out for some reassurance or assistance when overwhelmed with sadness
  – compensate for any nastiness, meanness and cruelty.
• They sink when:
  – feeling flat
  – emotionally drained
  – exhausted from trying to keep emotions in check
  – deflated from having had the wind taken from one's sails
  – the stuffing is knocked out of one
  – constantly displeased and critical of oneself and others.

The pancreas is at its best when the most is made of each and every opportunity.

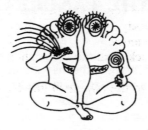

ALL WORK AND NO PLAY!

DEPENDING ON THE SPLENIC REFLEX

The splenic reflex is the small circular mound, on the upper outer quadrant of the left foot, which reflects stored hopes and dreams. It provides a solid base from which to test new ground vibrantly and enthusiastically whilst offering the uniformity and precision needed to get on. It monitors innermost feelings every time a corner is turned and, in so doing, gauges the influence of restraints that have become deeply ingrained, due to the many rules and regulations imposed by family and society when growing up. If too severe, these can put dampeners on many personal dreams. The need to do things in a certain way, whether it makes sense or not, in extreme situations can lead to obsessive behaviour; even though there is an innate knowing, deep down, that there is no one or 'right' way to do anything. The splenic reflex provides a good indication of the balance required.

- The splenic reflex swells:
  - when overly concerned, oversensitive or extremely particular about the way in which things should or should not be done
  - from having to stick to very strict rules and regulations, making it impossible to have a say in what is going on
  - due to obsessive tendencies
  - during a malarial attack from the indignation of having one's blood sucked.
- It flattens when going to the other extreme of:
  - no longer trying
  - being slovenly
  - not caring less.
- This reflex is adversely affected by the infamous 'disease to please'; one of the fastest-spreading epidemics of modern times, especially amongst law-abiding citizens, who take things to the extremes.

If being told what to do does not sit well, but there is a reluctant compulsion to do so anyway, then the spleen takes the brunt of it all. It can bring out the peevish, bad-tempered, piqued, mean, malevolent and spiteful side, which is enough to turn the blood, especially when unable to take any more. The feet can help to put the record straight and ensure that magnificent hopes and dreams do become a reality, no matter what the family and society say or think, provided the intent is good and the heart is in the right place.

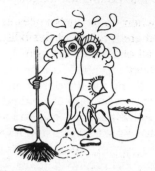

TIRED OF BEING TOLD WHAT TO DO.

FINDING THE ELBOW AND KNEE REFLEXES

The elbows and knees provide the flexibility to do all that is needed to make the most of every opportunity. Their reflexes are small bony protuberances, halfway along the outer edges of both feet, showing what is needed to fit in to emotional shifts whenever changing direction.

- The elbow reflexes jut out when:
  - elbowing one's way through life
  - resisting a change in direction
  - up to one's elbows
  - needing more space to get on...

...any one of which can affect hand movements.

- Hard skin forms over the elbow reflexes to:
  - protect any space that one does have
  - indicate the difficulty experienced in adapting to ongoing emotional changes.

Meanwhile the knees bend to fit into whatever is going on. Their primary reflexes are the same as those for the nipples, being in the middle of the balls of the feet, whilst their secondary reflexes are midway between the shoulder and elbow reflexes, roughly halfway down the balls of the feet on the outer edges. The latter are easier to 'read' when it comes to interpreting the language of the feet.

• These reflexes swell when up to one's knees in emotion.
• They protrude when there is a lack of flexibility, stubbornness or a resistance to change, all of which stem from:
  – a fear of being ridiculed
  – feeling inadequate
  – being terrified of losing control.
• Insubstantial-looking reflexes may be due to feeling weak-kneed.
• Hardened knee reflexes are a sign of being locked in obstinacy.

The elbows and knees provide the flexibility to go with the flow and to be open to all the many opportunities encountered on one's journey through life.

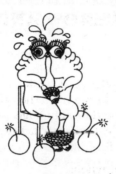

CAUGHT UP IN OTHER PEOPLE'S BUSINESS.

ALONG THE UPPER MIDDLE BACK REFLEXES

The bony ridges on the inner edges, that extend alongside the upper digestive reflexes, reflect the upper middle backbone. They reveal the backing and support when putting one's back into all that needs to be done, which either adversely or favourably affects future activities.

• The upper middle back reflexes distend and protrude when:
  – putting up such a resistance that it puts the back out

✳ 151

- a mound of disappointment, guilt and remorse gets in the way
- unable to achieve all that one sets out to do
- failing to meet certain expectations
- there is resentment at being walked over instead of bringing one's own brilliant ideas to the fore.
• These bony reflexes collapse due to:
  - pulling back instead of standing one's ground
  - the strain of being under tremendous pressure
  - constantly backing out or backing off
  - bending over backwards to please others
  - never being satisfied with the backing and support received.

Tension in the upper middle back almost instantaneously eases when assertively making one's innermost wishes known. This, part of the body has the ability to pivot, making it possible to see in every direction, except completely behind oneself, towards the past. However, the impact of prior experience can be seen on the opposite side of the upper digestive reflexes. Be aware of the following.

• Swellings over the upper middle back reflexes that come from the enormity of all that has been put behind one.
• The lower middle back reflexes collapse when:
  - breaking one's back
  - doing a great deal for little or nothing in return
  - feeling flat due to turning one's back on certain jobs.
• These areas become painful from:
  - the hurt of bending over backwards to please others, with little or no thanks, despite the pains gone to
  - the agony of shooting oneself in the foot
  - the discomfort of unfinished business or outstanding projects.
• Stiffness or rigidity in these parts could be from having the back against the wall or from being hard pressed to get things done.
• The bones pop up on top of the feet when pressurizing oneself.
• The tops of the feet become unusually cold when uncertain, scared or fearful due to inadequate backup.
• The arches of the feet burn with fury at the thought of all that went on, unknowingly, behind one's back.
• Hairs in these areas prevent ultra-sensitivity about what happened in the past.

When free of self-imposed restraints it's so much easier to weigh thing up and remain balanced.

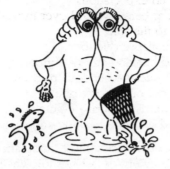

DROWNING FROM THE LACK OF SUPPORT.

TO SUM IT ALL UP

Feet are often on the receiving end of a barrage of abuse, especially during testing times; on top of which, they are frequently expected to take on weighty thoughts, as well as burdensome emotions that can really make things heavy going. Even though they do their level best to accommodate every whim and fancy, they do, from time to time, need to resort to changing their characteristics, especially when these hefty thoughts and emotions become noxious and a threat to personal well-being. Feet then highlight whatever is niggling beneath the surface in the hope that something is done to improve the situation. Images, initials, numbers and symbols (see page 107) are used to get the message across, and to provide insight as to how to deal with what's going on.

These necessary hindrances provide the ideal opportunity to get to know oneself better and to fix things in one's mind, knowing that much 'good' can come out of something that is seemingly 'bad'. It's by participating fully and taking complete responsibility for all that one does that the very best can be attained from life's circumstances.

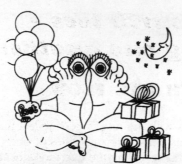

THE PRESENT IS A GIFT TO ONESELF.

TIP

Use the fiery nature of the third toes when massaging the feet to motivate and inspire. It really helps to get things going.

09 *The fourth toes – mirroring one another*

GOING WITH THE FLOW

The fourth toes, along with the ring fingers, reflect the more conservative, as well as non-conformist sides of one's personality, whilst, at the same time, revealing the need for a certain amount of routine, knowing that everything and everybody has its place. This is particularly important when bringing through unusual new concepts, when it is particularly necessary to be prepared for the unexpected. The fourth toes disclose the content or discontent of the mind regarding relationships, which either have a beneficial or detrimental effect on the chemical make-up of the body's secretions. Their agility indicates the amount of give and take within personal relationships, which, in turn, determines the flow of sensations and sensuality, helping one to stay in touch with oneself and others. These forthcoming toes provide an ongoing running commentary on anything that is upsetting within a relationship. The right fourth toe conveys the impact and impressions that prior unions have had whilst the left fourth toe reveals what's going on now within one's present liaisons. They are naturally supple and upright when true to their nature of being loving, accommodating and compassionate. Their lengths reveal the confidence of speaking up for oneself, whereas the size and shape of their toe pads display the capacity to be affectionate. Good communicators, such as writers, teachers, actors, broadcasters and so on, have noticeably large fourth toe pads but often need greater confidence and courage in bringing through extraordinary and different ways of communicating.

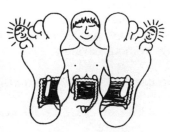

ENCOMPASSING LIFE.

GIVING IN TO OTHERS

When it comes to dealing with other people, the more approachable, honest and friendly one is, the better the fourth toes look. However, there are times when this does not happen with things that are being said or not said, heard or not heard, upsetting and having an impact on these toes. This, in turn, affects everything that enters or leaves the body.

- The fourth toes become unbending and rigid when:
  - highly principled, overly critical, extremely disapproving or unreasonably condemning
  - there are some very definite, non-negotiable views.
- They cringe and curl, making it difficult to face others:
  - when continuously brow-beaten
  - from being ridiculed and made a fool of
  - due to being unnecessarily submissive
  - when others keep taking advantage
  - because of distrust and defensiveness.
- A crooked fourth toe is a sign of:
  - going around the houses to explain things
  - not being absolutely direct and straight
  - using white lies or being intentionally deceitful.
- A squashed or boxed-in fourth toe occurs when:
  - withholding affection
  - choosing to be undemonstrative
  - being unable to relate to innermost feelings
  - keeping deep emotions well suppressed.
- Fourth toes bashfully bend across the third toes when:
  - thrown off track
  - constantly trying to please others
  - shy or lacking confidence
  - turning one's back on the family and society.
- Third toes overlap the fourth toes showing a preference for getting on and doing things without having to discuss the 'ins and outs' beforehand.
- Fourth toes overlap the third toes as a sign of 'all talk and no action'.
- Pressure from both sides may cause a ridge of hard skin down the centre of these toe pads from:

- not wishing to see the harsh realities of life
- viewing things from two completely different points of view, the family's and one's own.
- Hard skin covers the tips of the fourth toes when:
  - concealing intense irritability and frustration at not being able to communicate openly
  - there is extreme difficulty in getting amazing concepts out into the open.
- Corns appear on top of the fourth toes:
  - above the joints, to protect unique concepts and unusual ways of thinking
  - below the joints, to avoid getting it in the neck when opening the mouth.

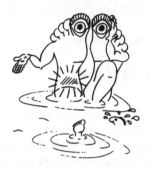

No energy for oneself.

In the lower halves of the instep

The lower halves of the insteps reveal whether anything worthwhile is being done with one's incredible new concepts and, if so, their effect on personal well-being. They mirror impressions left by other people's opinions, and reveal any impact on related organs reflected here, namely the small intestine, large colon, kidneys, fallopian tubes, uterus, ovaries, lower back and bottom halves of the upper arms and thighs. It's here, in the lower halves of the insteps, that the influence of all that which has been absorbed, mentally, emotionally, spiritually and physically, show up, with the lower half of the right instep conveying the residual effect of past relationships, whilst the left instep reveals the expectations of current liaisons. When smooth with no blemishes then it is a sign of going with the flow or having had many opportunities pass by with nothing meaningful happening.

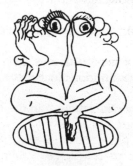

REBOUNDING BACK TO THE LOWER INSTEPS.

VICTIM OR VICTOR?

When things go wrong, there is the temptation to resort to victim mode, with a 'poor me' mentality of believing that nobody cares. Being fuelled by an en mass 'poverty consciousness' of never having enough, despite often having a great deal, doesn't help. The lack of energy and enthusiasm causes the lower halves of the insteps to sink, along with a heavy heart. Taking on the role of victim contaminates relationships as toxic words make things go from bad to worse. Utter despair can lead to self-destruction, with the denial and suffering of the body showing up on the feet in the hope that something worthwhile is done about it. The lower halves of the insteps reveal the impact of extreme emotions on personal communications and relationships.

- The lower halves of the insteps swell due to:
  - a buildup of noxious thoughts and dreadful emotions
  - feeling overwhelmed or smothered by others
  - drowning in self-pity.
- Undulations on the lower halves of the insteps indicate:
  - waves of anxiety from a fear of not being good enough
  - continual ups and downs within one's relationship.

- These areas look strained when:
  - tension with others has become unbearably strained
  - staying in an unhappy relationship for fear of having nothing else to move onto
  - feeling totally disempowered
  - locked in the past.
- Lines of concern reveal:
  - feeling tied down
  - concern about what others think and say
  - unwelcome ties to certain individuals.
- Scattered lines indicate:
  - being pulled in many directions
  - confusion regarding relationships
  - being left to put the pieces back together again.
- Flaking skin in these areas is a sign of extreme irritability with others getting on the nerves.
- Dry skin comes from:
  - giving more than required
  - extreme anxiety that wrings one dry
  - withdrawing into oneself
  - an insufficient exchange of ideas.
- Oedema is a sign of:
  - taking on far too much
  - hanging onto overwhelming emotive issues.
- An image of prison bars shows up when undergoing a life sentence of utter misery.
- Sweaty feet reveal extreme anxiety from not knowing what to say or how to say it, or from all that is heard or not being said.
- Red patches indicate anger at:
  - unreasonable expectations
  - having to sort something out that is best left alone
  - passionately trying to get an idea across.
- Yellow tinges reveal:
  - extreme discontent
  - feeling really fed up with certain people
  - a sunny disposition.
- White areas show:
  - a lack of energy
  - no interest in getting involved
  - divine guidance.

- Orange displays:
  - extreme annoyance at not being fully appreciated
  - a full range of emotions from extreme unhappiness to utter joy.

Overall, the lower halves of the insteps highlight how specific behaviour patterns and particular ways of speaking influence personal relationships.

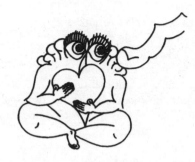

TRYING TO PLEASE, BUT GETTING NOWHERE.

AROUND THE SMALL INTESTINE REFLEXES

The small intestines are all about intimacy, as well as about being prepared to get up close and personal with one's own truth by being completely honest with oneself and others. It also reveals the willingness to go the whole nine yards, from the stomach to the colon, to sort out any nitty-gritty involved with getting to know others, especially during rough patches. This water-related tube relentlessly and continuously folds back and forth on itself as a way of getting to know all the ins and outs of every relationship, so that it knows who and what to take on board and who and what to leave alone. Its finger-like projections make sure that the very best can be gained from each and every encounter by dealing with all the finer details. By revealing the bigger picture there is then less of a temptation to jump in with both feet, even though every encounter, no matter how 'good 'or 'bad', is an ideal opportunity to find out more about oneself.

The small intestinal reflexes occupy the hollows on the lower halves of both insteps, from the waistlines of the feet to the heels, and reveal how ingrained beliefs and prior experiences interfere with the process of determining what is 'good' and what is 'bad'.

- The small intestine reflexes bulge when:
  - taking on too much
  - getting unnecessarily involved
  - having difficulty in communicating
  - feeling trapped within an unhealthy relationship.
- Ripples appear on the lower halves of the insteps due to:
  - being exceptionally unhappy and making waves
  - feeling really upset with all the ups and downs and comings and goings
  - things becoming extremely heavy going.
- Undulations that look more like ruts indicate being stuck in a rut.
- Scattered lines reveal:
  - utter confusion within personal relationships
  - not being able to take things in one's stride
  - having no direction.
- Lines that diagonally cross one another and look like netting or barbed wire are a sign of:
  - feeling entrapped
  - being in the midst of a conflict.
- Small intestine reflexes sink and look pale and drained whenever:
  - feeling overstretched and exhausted
  - in a relationship that saps one of energy.
- Wrinkles appear as a result of:
  - constant worry about making the same old mistakes
  - concern about what's being said or not said.

Every relationship is an ideal opportunity for ongoing personal development and is an essential part of the growth process, since it is through life's ups and downs that greater understanding of oneself is attained.

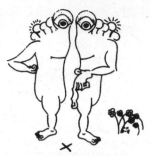

GETTING IN ONE'S OWN WAY.

GOING AROUND THE BEND

The fear of failure and having to face the ridicule that follows can be enough to drive people around the bend, especially when succumbing to the pressure of living in such a highly competitive society and being forced to go to such ridiculous extremes to prove oneself. Deep down, all anybody needs is recognition, appreciation and love for being unique. Difficulty in getting rid of the rougher, tougher aspects of life can lead to toxic relationships that contaminate the mind, body and soul. The large colon, therefore, does everything in its power to rid the body of endless loads of nonsense so that the mind and body don't get too bogged down.

All five sections of the colon are reflected onto the lower halves of both insteps, although they are not particularly clear to see. The ascending colon reflex climbs up the outer edge of the lower right instep as far as the waistline, where the hepatic reflex is situated, showing a willingness to release the remnants of the past. The transverse colon reflexes then extend across both insteps, just beneath the waistlines of both feet, curving slightly upwards, halfway along the left instep, to the splenic flexure reflex, to reveal the fine line between the past and present. Next the descending colon reflex follows the outer edge of the left lower instep, disclosing the ease of going with the flow. Finally, the sigmoid colon reflex backtracks along the top of the left heel to ensure that the residue of prior experiences passes on to the rectum and anus. The relief of letting go of the rougher aspects of life is symbolic of the relief of getting rid of the more toxic aspects of ongoing affiliations, whilst the bowel movement provides ample space in which to move on to the next stage.

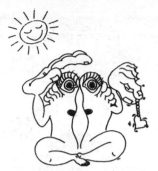

GETTING THE HEAD AROUND IT.

STUCK IN THE COLON

By eliminating the harsher aspects of life, the large colon clears the way for greater mental clarity, making sure that there is more energy for physical activities. With the remnants of the past out of the way, no more time or energy is wasted, which is why the colon is referred to as the generator of evolution and change. Should anything prevent it from transporting, transforming and eliminating surplus matter, then evidence of a perpetrator is likely to show up in the feet.

- The transverse colon reflexes swell when:
  - under tremendous pressure for all the wrong reasons
  - trying to meet unrealistically high expectations
  - being an absolute perfectionist
  - being hard on oneself
  - overcome with guilt about being out of control or feeling inadequate.
- These reflexes sink from:
  - giving in and feeling completely drained
  - being bulldozed or press-ganged into doing things against one's will to please others
  - feeling overwhelmingly disappointed at not meeting expectations.
- Colour plays a part so look out for:
  - red patches that indicate extreme anger at not being in control of the outcome, or passion
  - yellow areas of discontent or enlightenment within relationships
  - white parts that highlight absolute exhaustion from overwhelming demands or divine intervention

– bluish-black marks, which reveal emotional hurt and trauma, as
well as possible abuse.

Releasing past hurts, concerns and hardships before entering a new
relationship provides the opportunity to start afresh.

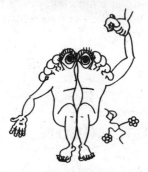

FEELING HELPLESS.

RUNNING THROUGH THE KIDNEYS

The kidney reflexes differ slightly from one another, with the left
kidney reflex being immediately below the left solar plexus reflex
(page 123) and the right reflex being fractionally lower and a little
more towards the arch. They reflect the ability to process life's events,
hanging onto anything that can be used again, whilst discarding
worked through thoughts and worn-out emotions that would
otherwise waste time and energy. When too many emotions
accumulate, the excess fluid in the body causes puffiness and
oedema. Too little water meanwhile dries the skin, making it flaky,
especially when feeling deserted or rejected. The kidneys are such an
emotional part of the body that they respond badly to being let
down, with any disillusionment or disappointment invariably bringing
out the thwarted 'kid' playing havoc with the 'kid-neys'. In extreme
circumstances, tantrums are likely. Many hurtful, resentful and
distressing memories reside in the kidneys, along with beliefs of being
badly neglected, abused or deprived. The unbearable pain of the past
makes its presence known in the back.

• The kidney reflexes sink when despondent, depressed or when
feeling drained.

- They swell with indignation and humiliation, when:
  – highly frustrated, extremely disappointed, excessively disillusioned
  – utterly dissatisfied with everything and everyone
  – feeling overwhelmingly let down.

To improve the situation the inner child needs to be loved and cherished, which then helps the body to remain composed and enjoy the very best composition.

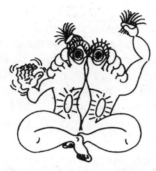

UNABLE TO FACE ANOTHER DISAPPOINTMENT.

CONCEPTS FROM THE OVARIES

Tiny 'water bubbles' that may be felt towards the outer edges of the feet are the ovarian reflexes and source of creation that participate in the formation of ongoing concepts and ideas. Meanwhile the womb reflexes, on the inner edges, where the insteps and heels meet, provide space for new beginnings to grow and develop. Sexual intimacy is the highest form of communication between two people, which is why the reproductive organs have such an important role to play when it comes to creating, nurturing and honouring new life, which then extends into one's relationships with one's chosen mate. Both types of sexual energy are present in males and females as a result of the parents' union, with the more dominant energy determining the characteristics. To visualize the female reproductive reflexes place the feet side by side. The fallopian tube reflexes stretch along the tops of the heels, showing where the male and female energies come together, before growing and developing, physically and metaphorically speaking. Meanwhile, the secondary fallopian tube reflexes extend over the tops of both feet, along the ankle creases, from the inner to the outer ankle bone.

- Hardness along the fallopian tube reflexes indicates a difficulty in bringing things together.
- Red strips over these reflexes reveal extreme frustration or anger when things don't happen as planned.
- White bands across them could be a sign of exhaustion from trying to force things.

Around the sixth week of pregnancy, a tiny embryonic-shaped reflex may be seen on one or other uterine reflex, but, if there are tiny bumps on both womb reflexes, then it could be twins. As soon as the baby's presence starts showing on the body, it usually shows up in the corresponding parts of the feet, either as shading or a swelling. Once the baby's head is engaged in the pelvis, a small round ball generally appears, near the bladder reflexes, on the insides of both feet.

- A cut between the womb reflexes and heels indicates:
  – the mother has cut herself off or feels cut off
  – severed ties with one's place of birth or family
  – a hysterectomy due to the woman feeling redundant and no longer of use to her family; sadness or resentment at no longer needing to nurture or provide a home; wishing to break free from the ties that come with being a woman.
- The womb reflexes look lifeless or hard, white and flat due to:
  – loss through miscarriage
  – a failed project
  – an aborted attempt at something new.
- A red womb reflex comes from extreme infuriation and frustration at not being appreciated.
- A red, puffy uterine reflex reveals anger at having one's femininity being taken advantage of, with endometriosis being a possibility.
- Broken blood vessels appear over these reflexes showing:
  – internal emotional wounds
  – physical trauma
  – some form of abuse.

The mother's womb is home for the first part of one's life, after which the body houses the mind and spirit and continues to do so for the remainder of one's life.

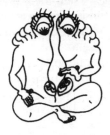

AT HOME WITH ONE'S SELF.

DOWN IN THE LOWER BACK

Along the bony inner edges, between the waistlines of the feet and the start of the heels, are the lower middle back reflexes, which support the individual's more substantial decisions and provide a firm basis upon which relationships are formed. The right foot reveals the after effects of prior relationships, first with one's parents and then with one's peers, whilst the left foot shows the consequences of current alliances with certain friends and colleagues, reinforced through the circumstances of one's partnerships. The lower back reflexes bring to the fore the reverse side of more impressionable relationships, revealing the more favourable or adverse affects. They also highlight the outcome of turning one's back on others, along with the accumulative effect of not having expectations met. Furthermore, this area is involved in decision making according to the impact of previous encounters.

- The lower middle back reflexes ache or swell:
  - with excruciating indecisiveness
  - when agonizingly caught between one's own needs and the requirements of others
  - due to feeling out of place, disorientated or unsupported, sometimes causing a disc to slip out of place.
- These reflexes are likely to sink, leaving one flat and deflated, when:
  - giving in to any undue pressure
  - having little or no energy to stand up for oneself
  - lacking the strength to confront others.

✴ 167

- The whole instep collapses when there is:
  - a complete breakdown in communications
  - a total lack of support within one's relationships
  - total devastation after a death, divorce, retrenchment and so on.
- Initials or numbers draw attention to:
  - anybody who has turned their back on them or vice versa
  - those who put one's back up
  - individuals who are fully behind you.
- Soreness across the tops comes from:
  - being really upset that others backed down after offering support
  - disappointment or disillusionment that affects the kidneys
  - getting it in the back for something that somebody else did.

The more the individual backs themselves, the more they find that others are behind them.

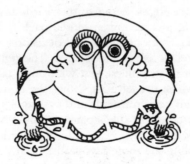

TRYING TO STAY AFLOAT.

A PAIR OF FEET

Feet are two of a kind! Or are they? Sometimes they are so different that they don't even look as though they belong to one another! As a pair they rely heavily on one another to get through life so, if one foot refuses to budge, the other can get hopping mad or bring things to a complete standstill. The right foot imparts the experiences and wisdom of the past, whilst the left foot is happy to be shown the way. In this way, prior circumstances provide the confidence to move forward, even though some fancy footwork may be required from time to time. However, this is far more preferable than dragging the feet and being held captive by the past. When there is resentment about the huge difference between past and present circumstances, it can make it difficult to maintain balance with the lack of coordination increasing the chances of tripping over one's own two feet. This can also happen when one foot desperately tries to get further ahead than the other. To stand one's ground and take stock of all that is going on feet need to work in unison, which is why the relationship of the pair is so important. Their relationship to one another provides valuable insight into one's relationship with oneself. Massaging both feet soothes things over and resolves outstanding issues so that both feet are steady and can waltz through life together.

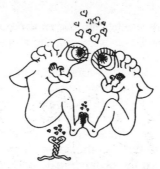

FEET STAND MIND, BODY AND SOUL IN GOOD STEAD.

FROM RIGHT TO LEFT

To remember what the right and left feet represent keep in mind the sayings 'you are dead **right**' and 'all that is **left** is the present'.

• The right foot reflects:
  – the right side of the body, which resonates to the past
  – the connection to ancestors and those who are older
  – the more masculine aspects of one's nature
  – past dealings, especially with men; one's father in particular
  – the influence of masculine opinions and beliefs
  – interaction with men in general.
• A tense right foot could indicate:
  – conflict in the past
  – ongoing uneasiness with one's own masculine traits.

- The left foot mirrors:
  - the left side of the body to show what is going on now
  - the impact of the present on the future
  - the link to everybody younger than oneself
  - the feminine side, exposing one's compatibility with women, especially the mother.
- A taut left foot is likely to be due to:
  - an unresolved disagreement with a woman or younger person
  - discomfort with one's femininity.

The body also gives clues as to which side is which since the liver stores memories and emotions from the past and is mainly on the right side of the body, reflected onto the right foot. Conversely, the bulk of the stomach is on the left side of the body and shows up on the left foot, with its reflexes revealing the ability to stomach life in the here and now

Other fascinating aspects to consider are that Universal energies are rapidly shifting from the male frequency of the Piscean era connected to the right foot, into the female vibrancy of the Aquarian age linked to the left foot. Also, with every step that is taken the left foot draws on the deep, mysterious and resourceful female energies derived from the earth through the soles. Conversely, the right foot attracts and pulls down the positive male energy of the sun, through the hairs on the head and body, throwing light on what happened in the past providing insight in the present

To keep moving through life, one foot is placed in front of the other, so that things can be worked out according to what happened in the past, which makes it easier to embrace and deal with the present.

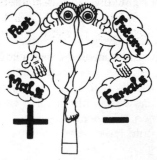

HAVING TO BE CONSTANTLY RIGHT UPSETS THE BALANCE.

DIFFERENCES BETWEEN THEM

For further insight, when looking at the right foot, also study the tops of the feet, since they reflect much of what happened in the past, which can help in understanding back problems. Meanwhile the left foot is energetically linked to the soles and all that is being confronted in the present, which is why, at times, the two can look so completely different. For instance, a strict upbringing, with little or no room to grow and develop, can stunt the development of both feet until, once free of restraints, they can start to grow accordingly. That is unless the horror of the past holds the right foot back, whilst the left foot takes full advantage of the freedom in the present. Feet generally show their differences through discrepancies in their size, shape, colour or condition, so aspects to look for are listed below.

- General tension coming from:
  - an overall resistance to life
  - holding back for fear of moving forward.
- A heavier right foot is usually weighed down by unresolved emotions of the past.
- A heavier left foot reveals the burdens of the here and now.
- A larger right foot indicates greater independence previously.
- A larger left foot is indicative of breaking free from prior restraints.
- A smaller left foot is constrained by current circumstances.
- A smaller right foot hangs on to the shackles of the past.
- The right foot becomes misshapen when:
  - unreasonable beliefs distort its development
  - there is a misinterpretation of what went on whilst growing up.
- A misshapen left foot is likely to be disfigured by:
  - constantly trying to fit into unsuitable beliefs
  - succumbing to unbelievable pressure now.

The need to always be right can leave one left out in the future!

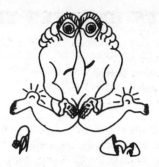

THE FUTURE IS NOT WHAT IT USED TO BE.

TIP

Rubbing feet releases the mind from the grips of fear and allows the body to let go of frightful memories, which gives the odds the opportunity to even themselves out.

ABOVE THE ELBOWS AND OVER THE KNEES

The ability to embrace fully those who come and go in one's life, yet be able to move on, all the wiser yet unburdened, shows up on the lower halves of the upper arms and thighs. The reflexes for these extend along the outside edges of both feet, showing the ease with which the arms open to hug others and bring them closer to the heart, according to how good one feels about oneself. A reluctance to do so, by keeping others at arm's length, avoids the need to get too close, either physically or emotionally. So it is that these parts of the arm symbolically represent the acceptance or rejection of oneself, which then influences the way in which life is handled. Difficulty in doing so provides the ideal opportunity to find an amicable way for everybody to be happy.

- The reflexes for the lower halves of the upper arms swell when:
  – important relationships stagnate
  – feeling desperately out of control emotionally.
- These reflexes collapse when:
  – tired of carrying heavy loads
  – emotionally exhausted
  – there is no longer the strength to reach out.

Meanwhile the lower portions of the thighs assist the legs in working well. They take on the whole body, as well as immense emotional burdens that can come with it. In so doing, they provide incredible inner strength, along with the wherewithal of when to let go. If something dreadful happened in a past relationship then there could be a fear of opening up too much. Extra fat acts as a form of protection. The thigh reflexes can then look overwhelmed or utterly exhausted. The more open one is the less judgemental one becomes.

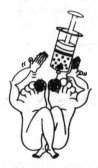

GIVING OTHERS THE WRONG IDEA.

WHEN ALL IS SAID AND DONE

Communication, vital for personal growth, is the means by which each individual develops their own individuality and gets to know themselves and others better. Every thought and each word has a specific vibration that can have a destructive or constructive outcome, depending on the passion instilled into them. With so many different roles being played daily, the behaviour and script changes accordingly. It is what is said, along with the way in which it is said, that makes every relationship so very different. For instance, close friends are treated differently to perfect strangers; until the stranger becomes a friend. Yet weariness towards the stranger part of oneself is due to compromising values and adapting unique qualities to suit parents, then teachers, peers, colleagues and so on, to such an extent that the individual becomes a stranger to themselves. Not trusting others makes it difficult to make friends with oneself! Yet the solution is simply to be oneself! As respect grows between individuals, so too does harmony both inside and outside the body.

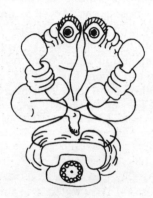

ENJOYING A GOOD RELATIONSHIP WITH ONE'S SELF.

10 The little toes – facilitating progress through life

THE MOBILE TOES

The earth-like qualities of the little toes, along with those of the little fingers, provide a firm foundation and a fair amount of flexibility to think for oneself. Being on the outer edges of both feet, these toes anchor and ground personal thoughts for ongoing growth, development and progress. At the same time, they provide mental agility, constant alertness and ongoing awareness of all the amazing opportunities that come along. The little toes support change and evolvement encouraging the expansion of the mind. In this way unique ways of thinking can develop. Being a maverick can get one in trouble from time to time, yet taking risks is essential for progress. These toes reveal patience, dependability and consideration, all of which stem from a long line of ancestors. They reflect one's roots and reveal the impact of inherent family and social beliefs that, if out-dated, can either hold one back or drive one to despair. They confirm that there is no need to follow in another's footsteps since everybody is meant to be different.

These toes vibrate to red, the lowest colour vibration and are strongly connected to the solidarity of the skeletal system, the flexibility of the muscular system, the ongoing movement of the excretory system, along with the endless possibilities of the reproductive system. When mobile and upstanding they reveal individuality, with their lengths showing the degree of confidence when it comes to speaking up for oneself within the family and society. Meanwhile the size and shape of the little toe pads demonstrate the capacity to think outside the box, which unleashes the spirit and allows one to be oneself.

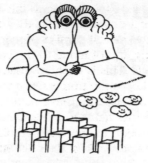

FREE TO SOAR!

NOTE

There was once a great deal of superstition around sixth toes, which meant that giving birth to a baby with extra digits was a really terrifying and highly disgraceful experience; so much so that the baby was immediately taken away and usually drowned. Today these toes are generally removed surgically, after which there is little or no mention of them because of the stigma that is still attached to them. Yet their positions, next to the little toes, on the outer edges of both feet, immediately points to extraordinary concepts that do not fit in or conform to the norm, which seems to pose such a threat to society. However, these innovative ideas are desperately needed for human evolvement. The good news is that even when physically removed, the energy of these incredible concepts remains and can be drawn upon at any time to add extra dimensions to thoughts and ideas.

MOULDING THE LITTLE TOES

Over the years the characteristics of the little toes become moulded into a variety of shapes and sizes. First comes the influence of family and society, then pressure from one's peers, followed by the expectations of colleagues at work and various partners throughout life, with the eventual possible responsibility of bringing up children.

The little toes are fashioned according to the amount of dependence, independence and inter-dependence, as they adapt to often diverse beliefs. They reveal the mental conflict of trying to conform to out-dated ways of thinking and of trying to pretend to be the person that everybody else expects. This is likely to distort their shape and squash them, which keeps the true essence locked within, even though it's contrary to one's inquisitive nature. Asking the individual to describe their little toes helps to understand their perception of themself and their position in life. Keep in mind that the right little toe reveals their past status, whilst their left little toe symbolizes their current circumstances.

- When the little toes are barely visible from underneath it could be due to:
  - concealing one's own true thoughts
  - being highly sensitive
  - being concerned about what others think.
- The little toes curve and fall over themselves when:
  - succumbing to the family's way of thinking that are alien to one's own
  - giving in to unreasonable social conditioning.
- These toes hide behind the fourth toes because of being:
  - too frightened to be oneself
  - limited by self-imposed restrictions.
- The little toes look insignificant when:
  - feeling unimportant in the greater scheme of things
  - constantly putting oneself down
  - family pressure stunts growth, physically and metaphorically.
- They hold back because of:
  - needing to move on but being reluctant to do so
  - extreme fearfulness in dealing with family issues.
- These toes become rigid when:
  - so obsessed with physical possessions that it stamps out individuality
  - accumulated wealth is believed to be the only way to find security
  - there's a resistance to becoming the person others expect one to be.

The little toes come into their own when there is the courage to stand out from the crowd and the individual is true to themselves no matter what.

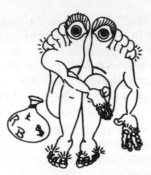

AFFECTING SELF WORTH.

NOTE

If the little toes constantly move whilst the feet are being massaged then it is a sign of wishing to break free from family and social constraints and be oneself.

SMALL BUT STRONG

Of all the toes, the little toes are bashed around the most when swaying from side to side and refusing to commit one way or another. They take the brunt of the weary mind when there's a reluctance to succumb to the family's or society's way of thinking, yet feeling resentful about being caught up anyway.

- The little toes look restrained and may even end up leaning against the fourth toes for additional support when hard pressed for a solution.
- They can look bashed when jumping in with both feet and being ruthlessly criticized.
- These toes turn in when:
  - constantly trying to keep the peace
  - turning one's back on the futility of all the nonsense.
- A ridge of hard skin down their centres is a sign of:
  - being prevented from seeing or getting involved with the greed, scepticism and pessimism of modern society, especially when having different and less harsh views

– keeping oneself to oneself.
- The little toes choose to stand alone when:
  – feeling like an outsider
  – severing dependence on the family
  – wishing to be recognized as an individual.
- The little toe may break when desperate to break free and be oneself.
- A bent little toe reveals:
  – a troubled or overburdened soul
  – taking on more than necessary
  – trying to constantly please the family.
- Red little toes are a sign of:
  – being embarrassed about others seeing through one
  – anger at being manipulated.
- These toes look pale and white when:
  – drained by unreasonable family or social demands
  – extremely spiritual.
- They turn blue:
  – from the hurt of having to conform whether one likes it or not
  – when needing to give voice to one's own way of thinking.
- Corns on the outside edges, over the ear reflexes, appear when:
  – not wanting to hear what's going on, especially within the home
  – constantly turning a deaf ear because of what was said in the past
  – protecting oneself from hearing the same old thing over and over again.

These toes love it when individuals venture out and are different.

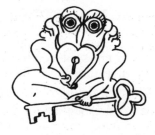

THEY HOLD THE KEY TO INDIVIDUALITY.

DOWN AT THE HEELS

Heels symbolize the freedom and space to be oneself, with their earthly qualities ensuring that personal concepts have a good base and are grounded. They resonate to red, which ensures ample energy to keep moving and make progress, as well as the strength and determination to keep going through life's ups and downs. Meanwhile their cushion-like structures bolster and support mind, body and spirit every step of the way, offering the security and freedom needed to expand and make the most of every situation. This, in turn, strengthens the skeletal system and keeps the muscles agile and well toned, which is important when it comes to letting go of the past and ensuring that the excretory organs are in good condition. Once the way is clear, then new concepts and ideas can be generated in the hope that something worthwhile is done with them; this helps to keep the reproductive system in top form. The heels epitomize the opposames. For instance, they display the need to be strong yet gentle; they know when to expand and when to hold back; to release yet embrace; to honour the masculine, as well as the feminine traits, yet remain unique. As they do so, they ensure constant evolvement and transformation, preventing the human species from becoming extinct.

Reflected onto the heels is the pelvis, along with the lower excretory and reproductive glands and organs, plus the bulk of the skeletal and muscular system. The hip reflexes are on the outer ankle bones, below which are the feet and buttock reflexes in the curves of the heels, whilst the hand reflexes are the small mounds in front of the outer ankles. Within the small triangular area, immediately beneath the inner ankle bones, are the internal reflexes of the anus, rectum, bladder, along with the prostrate gland and penis on males, and the uterus and vagina on females. Being such a multidimensional being with many facets can, at times, be confusing, so it helps to trust the process and relish, as well as learn from, the ongoing adventures of life. Further exciting encounters can bring enrichment and knowledge as one ventures into the unknown and discovers virgin territories.

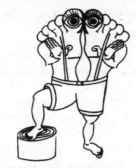

OVERCOMING BLOCKAGES.

DIGGING THE HEELS IN

A balanced and healthy approach to life keeps the heels pliable and provides a spring in the step, with the right heel showing the ability to progress in the past; whilst the left heel reveals current developments. Should the burden of emotional responsibilities get too great then the heels are likely to become a drag and drag their way through life, making it difficult to put one foot in front of another. Other aspects to consider include the following.

- Hefty heels show that life is heavy going because of:
  - immense commitments to the family and society
  - feeling down at the heels
  - being prevented from moving ahead.
- Swollen heels indicate:
  - feeling bogged down by the trivialities of life
  - being overwhelmed by responsibilities
  - a belief that the future is bleak.
- A spare tyre around the edges indicates:
  - feeling as though one is drowning
  - wallowing in self-pity
  - needing extra security
  - requiring an extra boost because of feeling so flat
  - an inadequate support system
  - safeguarding one's manhood or womanhood from abuse.
- Broad heels reveal a solid foundation from which to move, but when they are too big they can be a hindrance, causing one to laboriously ponder over the wasteful aspects of life.

★ 181

- Narrow heels are a sign of having to tread carefully so as to:
  - not disturb the peace
  - avoid attracting attention in an already fraught family situation
  - remain unnoticed until taking to one's heels.
- Hard skin develops around the heels when:
  - feeling especially vulnerable
  - no longer wishing to be taken advantage of
  - needing to survive and get through harsh times
  - there are lower back problems
  - digging the heels in and refusing to budge
  - compensating for feeling deeply insecure
  - wanting to get ahead no matter what.

Some women believe it to be a precaution against falling pregnant and, if it works for them, so be it!

- Flaking skin in these areas indicates extreme irritation at the lack of progress.
- If it flakes over the hard skin, then there is likely to be exceptional frustration at having to constantly protect one's every move.
- The heels crack up from:
  - being pulled in many different directions
  - feeling divided as to which way to turn
  - being torn apart by conflicting views.

Massaging the heels with a good dollop of heel balm helps to centre and ground the soul, making way for greater inner peace and a more focused direction.

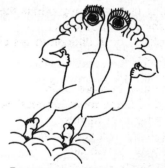

REFUSING TO BUDGE.

HOT ON THE HEELS

The high incidence of heel disorders comes from extreme uncertainty with so many being falsely lured and imprisoned in a materialistic and money-orientated society.

- A spur, like an anchor, holds one back:
  - from the foot incessantly being put down
  - because of constantly wanting things in certain limited ways
  - due to the agony of trying to get ahead.
- Painful heels come from wishing to move on yet reluctant to take the first step.
- Growing pains reveal the difficulty in being oneself, making:
  - the whole growing up experience extremely torturous
  - anything to do with sexuality being an absolute pain.
- Bruised heels are from kicking the heels due to being hurt or anxious about the direction of one's life, especially when prevented from moving on.
- Burning heels come from:
  - the blood boiling because of not being able to get ahead
  - feeling furious about current circumstances.
- Cold heels reveal a lack of confidence and enthusiasm to get going.
- Blistered heels indicate:
  - incessant friction in the family
  - being rubbed up the wrong way.
- Shiny heels indicate:
  - feeling worn out from endless conflict and resistance
  - being a shining light, showing others the way
  - taking on a shine of one's own.
- Spongy heels often find it difficult to get ahead showing:
  - constant indecision
  - congestion from fear
  - a tendency to give in more easily
  - the likelihood of being more impressionable.
- Heels wrinkle whenever there's:
  - concern that things will get in the way
  - worry about what lies ahead
  - anxiety about safety and security.
- Rippled heels are a sign of being stuck in a rut from the monotony of doing the same old thing time and time again.

- Black marks on the heels usually indicate deep prejudice.
- The Achilles bone becomes prominent when the journey through life is believed to be an uphill journey with a lot to overcome along the way.

It takes great courage to release oneself from out-dated and unrealistic social constraints, but it is the only way in which to embark on the journey of self-discovery. The pain, frustration, stress, resentment and so on, experienced en route, provide the opportunity to work things out, so that healing can take place, and the spirit be set free so that it can then soar and attain unbelievable heights.

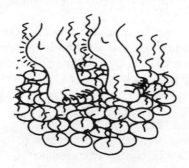

HOT ON THE HEELS.

AT THE HIP REFLEXES

Hips provide the 'umph' needed to thrust ahead, which is why, when stepping forward with confidence, towards something that is worth striving for, the hips are supple and free. They provide the strength to haul the whole body over anything that comes along, with the option to change direction at any time. Innately everybody needs to feel useful and know that they are doing something worthwhile since this provides the much-needed impetus to stay motivated. The hips also help to ground the energy so that the mind, body and spirit are in the best possible position to take a stand. Problems only arise when losing sight of personal dreams or when giving up on oneself because of feeling hopeless, lost and bewildered.

- Puffy hip reflexes show:
  - inner resentment at being stripped of dignity and self-worth
  - that life is heavy-going

– difficulty in standing up for oneself.
- Swollen hip reflexes indicate:
  – extreme dissatisfaction
  – exceptional fear.
- Miniscule broken veins on the hip reflexes reveal exceptional sadness at the course that one's life has taken.

Realizing how amazing it is to have survived so many hardships, yet to still be standing, makes it so much easier to honour and appreciate oneself. These experiences can be used to inspire oneself as well as others.

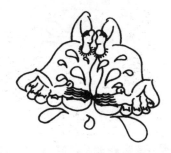

WHEN LIFE GETS TO BE A LITTLE TOO MUCH.

FINALLY LETTING GO

Letting go of fearful memories and en mass hysteria that reside in the heart and body is extremely liberating, making it then possible to walk one's talk and speak one's truth. The way in which the body does this is through the release of urine, faecal matter, wind and sweat, all of which provide an outlet for worked-through thoughts and unwanted emotions. This relieves the mind and body of hidden guilt complexes, inexplicable traumas and unresolved conflicts that are generally lugged around for longer than necessary. If these are retained, they could become highly toxic and extremely harmful to personal well-being, which is picked up by the reflexes for the excretory system, namely the urethra, rectum and anus. These are all on the inner triangular parts of the heels, although the bladder reflexes are the small bulges on the insides of both feet, situated where the insteps and heels meet.

- The bladder reflexes swell quite noticeably when:
  - there's difficulty in letting go
  - unresolved issues get in the way
  - distressed about the conflict with one's partner.
- Small broken blood vessels on the inside of ankles reveal extreme unhappiness at having to put up with so much nonsense that wastes time and energy.

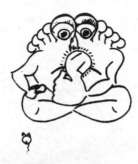

THE THUMB'S UP TO MOVE ON.

THE ART OF REPRODUCTION

The reproductive glands and organs constantly fill the mind, body and soul with renewed energy for ongoing expansion, as well as the reproduction of fantastic concepts for the benefit of society as a whole. The male input encourages new liaisons to take place, whilst the female energy supplies a safe space and harmonious environment in which resultant unions can grow and develop. All of this is reflected on the small triangular areas on the insides of both heels, alongside the lower excretory reflexes. The position of the testes reflexes varies according to weather conditions; hanging around the tips of the inside heels when it's warmer, and migrating up towards the insteps as it gets cooler. Unusual reflexes are listed below.

- Broken blood vessels over the reproductive reflexes reveal:
  - deep unhappiness at being taken advantage because of one's gender
  - sadness at not being fully appreciated.

- Pain in this part of the heel indicates:
  - extreme hurt at not receiving the recognition that one believes to be deserved.
  - possible difficulty in rising to the occasion because of feeling unimportant, increasing the chances of being impotent.
- The reproductive reflexes often sink when tired of having to do everything because of one's gender.
- Swollen reflexes are a sign of reaching out to be noticed for who and what one is.
- White lumps and bumps are pockets of contained anger and frustration that are gender related.

Children bring immeasurable gifts of greater understanding through the challenges that they present. They mirror those aspects of the parents that still need addressing.

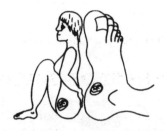

USE EVERY OPPORTUNITY TO CREATE SOMETHING SPECIAL.

On to the Buttock Reflexes

The outer triangles of the heels contain the reflexes for the buttocks which, as the seat of power, provide all the basic backup needed. Problems arise when there are memories of any unpleasantness that 'went on down there', which is still a pain in the butt. This causes these reflexes to act as a sore reminder of many injustices and unfair punishments.

- The buttock reflexes turn black and blue from:
  - extreme hurt
  - injured pride

- constant hidings
- a bum deal.
- The buttock reflexes become tense due to:
  - traumatic memories of being potty trained making it difficult to be spontaneous
  - refusing to let go
  - having a firm hold on the purse strings
  - taking on the role of victim.
- The heels swell when:
  - somebody is being a 'pain in the bum'
  - there are painful and hurtful memories of being powerless
  - feeling bogged down.

The buttocks are right behind one when it comes to taking back one's power and being fully responsible for the circumstances of one's own life.

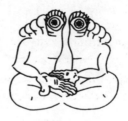

LIFE CAN BE A REAL PAIN IN THE BUTT!

IN THE LOWER BACK

Around the C-shaped ridges of the inner ankle bones are the lower back reflexes, which reveal the solidarity and basic support believed to come from financial backing. Feeling strong and valuing oneself strengthens the lower back, which then provides the flexibility and agility to make progress. Since this is where the will resides, there is the ongoing opportunity to become more of oneself and, in so doing, enhance one's self-worth. Failure to do so adversely affects the lower back and shows up in its reflexes. A lot of discontent can accumulate here, often making it a really troublesome area, made worse when feeling deeply insecure or when concerned about finances. Anything that is a pain and gets in the way of progress can result in lower back problems, affecting the overall movements. If tension builds up here, it can impinge on the nerves in the leg causing them to ache or even become numb if the pain is so bad that there is a subconscious desire to no longer feel it. In extreme situations, the legs can become paralyzed with fear.

- The lower back reflexes swell when:
  - reaching out for greater recognition and validation, generally in the form of financial reward
  - needing to get a move on.
- These reflexes become engorged when:
  - disillusioned and worried
  - relying too heavily on materialism.
- The lower back reflexes collapse because of:
  - insufficient inner resources to draw on
  - not having the power to do what one really needs to do
  - feeling out of control
  - a lack of finances backing one up
  - exhaustion from carrying around hefty thoughts and derogatory emotions.

Backing oneself, every step of the way, allows the lower back to follow suit, so that every experience enriches and empowers the true spirit.

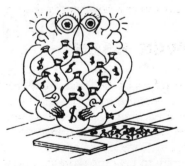

IT'S TIME TO APPRECIATE ONESELF.

UP IN THE ARMS AND AT THE TOP OF THE THIGHS

Also connected to the little toes and heels, and linked to personal security and mobility, are the top parts of the upper arms and thighs. These reflexes are either side of the feet, with the upper arm reflexes in the feelings area, along the edges of the balls of the feet, whilst the thigh reflexes are further along, in the communion areas. The former reflexes reveal the strength and flexibility behind a wide range of hand movements, and highlight heartwrenching feelings that are emotionally out of control or helplessly beyond reach. Meanwhile, the upper halves of the thighs, associated with sexuality, are subconsciously influenced by the parent's approach and their views on sexual matters. The more open the thighs, the greater the openness to anything new, whereas holding the thighs tightly together is often an unconscious way of protecting sexuality. Thigh issues may result from unresolved parental problems, traumatic childhood memories, deep hurts and the inability to express true desires, any of which can play havoc with the reproductive hormones, as well as approach to sexuality. Just by feeling good helps the acceptance of oneself and others.

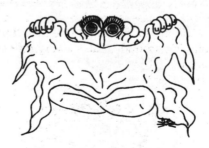

OPENING UP TO ALL POSSIBILITIES.

SIZING UP THE FEET

The feet size things up according to how the individual measures up to others, as well as measures others up. Their size can change, so much so that there are times when they can end up being proportionately different. Their dimensions can diminish if there's constant belittlement and severe social constraints. Also, constantly withdrawing and holding back, because of misinformation continually being advertised and bantered about, limit the body, hamper the soul and clamp down on the feet. Even though there can be often a deep desire to break free from these restraints, the fear of being ostracized is so great that many downsize to fit in, even though there can be resentment from being forced to do this. Any form of limitation reduces the size of the feet, whilst breaking free from social restrictions allows them to embrace their full size.

When it comes to reading the feet, first ask the individual whether they are happy with the size of their feet. If they think that they are too big, inquire 'too big for what?' If they believe them to be too small, then question what being 'too small' means to them. This helps in determining the steps needed to balance things out. When the feet are two different sizes, compare the circumstances of the past and the present to get the full measure of the feet. When comfortable with the size of one's feet it's easier to make a favourable impression every time the foot is put down. Any impression made by the feet depends on its physical mass, as well as the way in which it is placed on the ground, according to the mood one is in. For instance, stamping and stomping around creates a very different impression to pussyfooting around.

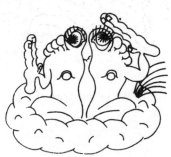

UP AGAINST ONESELF.

Language of the Feet

The size of the feet can reveal a side that is often kept out of sight since it can show how impressionable one is, along with some very sizeable information.

- Larger feet have a far greater surface with which to impress and be impressed.
- The bulk of the feet determines the size of the impression made.
- Their substance reveals the ability to reach one's full potential.
- If the feet are too large there's a tendency to keep putting one's foot in it and get nowhere fast.
- Feet that are too big for their boots are a sign of being bigheaded or outgrowing the past.
- Smaller feet are just as capable of making a big impact but the chances are that:
  - there's a reluctance to attract too much attention
  - they prefer others not to know what they are up to
  - there's a need to tread carefully
  - the ground is cautiously tested before making up one's mind
  - they hold back despite missing out on the greater scheme of things.

When assessing the size of feet, also take into consideration their width since this reveals their willingness to conform.

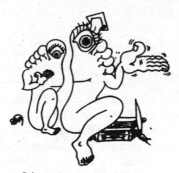

IT'S BEST TO BE YOURSELF.

> **NOTE**
>
> The size of the feet constantly changes, even throughout adulthood. The more ground that is covered, the bigger the feet; whereas constantly holding back will make them shrink, since they are not being used to their full potential, either physically or metaphotically. All this can change and as it does so, so too do the feet!

CRIPPLING THE BODY

Society has reached such an intolerable level of pain, despair and fear that many have forgotten who they really are, which then prevents them from being completely honest, truthful or loyal to themselves, let alone to other people. A huge chunk of life is based on mistruths, with cover-ups being constantly used so as not to be seen to be stepping out of line. This prevents individuals, as well as their family and friends, from getting to know the true self, resulting in incredible mistrust and extreme insecurity. Not only does it make it difficult to get ahead, but also holds back the whole family, as well as colleagues, friends and so on. It's little wonder that there is so much unease, disease and crime in the world today!

At the root of it all is fear. Fear has gained such a firm foothold that it has virtually taken over, despite many no longer knowing what they are fearful of! To compensate, inbuilt emotional defence mechanisms are developed and rigid belief systems constructed in a desperate attempt to survive in a highly critical, social environment. Compounding this dreadful state of affairs is the fact that society has become highly achievement-orientated; there is an immense amount of frustration, incredible resentment and terrible bewilderment. To cope, things are done faster, but not always better, with the pressure becoming so emotionally and spiritually crippling that disease is inevitable. Making the situation worse is the fact that most people have become so secure with their insecurity that they don't want to change, even though it stunts their growth, along with national and global development. The greatest crime is not being true to oneself but, fortunately, it is never too late to bring all this to an end, with tremendous opportunities lying at the feet.

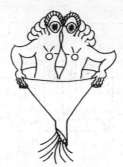

THERE'S NO NEED TO FIT IN.

STRIVING TO BE FREE

Worldwide freedom and peace is possible once everybody has the courage to free themselves emotionally and spiritually from the dreadful social restraints and political constraints. By changing oneself, a part of the world changes, giving others the courage to do the same. To help to bring crime and disease to an end we should try to do the following.

- Stop feeding the fear and 'victim mentality'; instead focus on the good in life.
- Stop trying to meet other people's expectations; instead focus on making a valuable contribution by being different.
- Stop robbing yourself or others of amazing opportunities; instead focus on what the soul came to do.
- Stop allowing others to take advantage; instead focus on doing something really worthwhile.
- Stop emotionally hijacking yourself by criticizing others; instead focus on being unique.

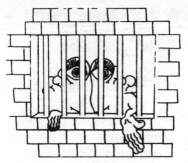

BREAK FREE FROM SELF-IMPOSED RESTRAINTS.

TEN TOP TIPS

Instead of focusing on money for all the wrong reasons, see it as an energy from which everybody can prosper and draw in to their life. Try to remember the following:

1 Appreciate everything and everybody.
2 Pay interest in all that is done.
3 Give credit to oneself and others.
4 Treasure precious moments.
5 Enjoy good fortune.
6 Put the best into everything.
7 See everything as worthwhile, profitable and beneficial.
8 Value every experience as an enriching one.
9 Know that everybody is worth the effort.
10 Believe in the abundance of life.

Wealth can only bring happiness when enrichment is enjoyed on all levels.

11 On top of the feet – exposing the past

GOING ON IN THE BACKGROUND

Although portions of the tops of the feet have already been covered, there are some useful generalizations to consider, such as whether these areas are flexible, strong and lively enough to back every thought, feeling, action, reaction and relationship and provide sufficient security and confidence to face life full on. It all depends on what went on in the past, and what has been put behind one. Most of the secondary reflexes are situated here and show what goes on at the back of the organs, since this is where hurtful memories and inhibiting beliefs are tucked away when too terrifying to deal with. The tops of the feet, therefore, relay information regarding the reverse or shadow side and, in so doing, reveal whatever it is that is holding one back or whether anything untoward is going on in the background.

- From the tops of the big toes, along the inside edges of the feet, to the tips of the heels, are the intellectual boundaries which substantiate and back up unique notions.
- From the tips of the second toes to the ankle creases are the parts that reveal inner confidence.
- The strips that extend from the tips of the third toes to the ankle creases show the support given to personal concepts.
- From the tips of the fourth toes to the ankle creases are the parts that display the effect of interactions with others.
- From the tips of the little toes, along the outer edges of the feet, to the end of the heels are the social and family boundaries that reveal the ability to expand from the tried and tested and move on.

The tops of the feet reflect the back and vibrate to every colour, as well as each of the elements.

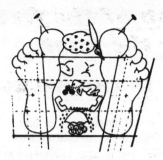

PROVIDING FULL SUPPORT.

OUTER BOUNDARIES

The outer edges of the feet form an essential part of the framework for the body. Their position allows them to offer a certain amount of security and also an outline of what's going on, so that decisions can be made regarding the next move. The bulk of the limbs are reflected on the sides of the feet in the hope that life is embraced and experienced to the full, which is so much easier with a relaxed approach. Even though tripping and stumbling from time to time is inevitable, the important thing is to have the confidence to pick oneself up, dust oneself down and keep on going. The limbs are depicted as follows.

- In the arm reflexes:
  - the socket of the arms are the prominent bones beneath the little toes
  - the upper arm reflexes (page 190) extend along the outer edges of the balls of the feet
  - the elbow reflexes (page 150) are the small bones halfway along
  - the lower arm reflexes (page 144) veer up from here at a 45 degree angle
  - the hand reflexes (page 67) are soft mounds in front of the outer ankle bones.
- In the leg reflexes:
  - the hip reflexes (page 184) are on the outer ankle bones
  - the thigh reflexes (page 190) stretch from the outer ankle bones to the midway points above the upper arm reflexes

★ 197

- the knee reflexes (page 150) are where the thigh reflexes end
- the shin reflexes (page 114) double back on themselves and then follow the outer edges of the feet as far as the start of the heels
- the feet reflexes (page 167) are immediately beneath the outer ankle bones.

Changes of characteristics to look out for include the following.

- The limb reflexes swell whenever:
  - wishing to break free, especially from social restraints
  - needing more space.
- These reflexes sink or flatten when:
  - giving in to social or family pressure
  - breaking under the strain.

The outer edges of the feet show the amount of freedom the individual believes that they have to spread their wings and fly. As they grasp their reason for being they can gain so much more from each leg of their journey through life.

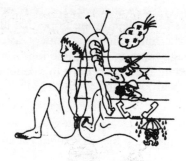

ON THE SIDE.

IN THE CENTRE OF THE BODY

The narrow strips along the fleshy insteps, beneath the bony arches, reflect the central organs of the body and represent the core of one's being, revealing the substance one is made of. To understand this better, imagine the body sliced in half and then superimpose the divided organs onto the fleshy insteps. The right instep carries the impressions of the past, whilst the left instep mirrors the impact of what's going on inside now.

- Between the upper and lower surfaces of the big toes are the reflexes for the segments of the brain, pituitary and pineal glands, as well as nasal and mouth cavities, from which greater insight can be gained into innermost thoughts.
- Along the toe necks, the reflexes for the slit larynx, pharynx and thyroid gland give an inside story on the exchanges that take place.
- Down the inner edges of the balls of the feet are the sliced apart reflexes for the windpipes and oesophagus, along with the thymus gland and heart, which reveal deep feelings.
- The upper halves of the fleshy part of the insteps contain the reflexes for the chopped-apart fundus of the stomach, the pancreas and jejunum, displaying a gut feel of what is being done.
- The rest of the fleshy insteps reveal the divided portions of the large and small intestinal reflexes, giving the low down on what's going on at a deeper level within relationships.
- The triangular portions on the inner heels carry the reflexes for the split-apart bladder, lower reproductive organs, rectum and anus, and disclose the harmony and security within.

The arches help determine how to bridge the gap between what happened in the past and what can be done now to improve the situation.

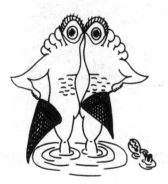

TRAPPED IN BETWEEN.

HELP FROM THE INSIDE OUT

Feet take one on a journey that covers many terrains, from the plateaus of pleasure to the deserts of loneliness; from oceans of love to jungles of entrapment; from peaks of success to deep canyons of failure; from highways of happiness to low roads of sorrow. The road for today came from yesterday's journey and is en route to tomorrow's mystery tour. So, even though it is possible to stay in 'yesterday' or go quickly into 'tomorrow', it does mean missing out on today's journey. When a path is chosen with love, then it's possible to make the most of every step by following one's heart and planting seeds of brilliance along the way. The most impressionable and worthwhile footprints can then be left in the sands of time, as the calling cards of one's life. On this journey of self-discovery one gets to know oneself better by visiting parts of oneself that have never been explored before. Should life, at any stage, become stagnant or seem to be going nowhere, then the heart is the best place to go to for directions. The journey on earth is intentionally filled with endless challenges to test temperance and resourcefulness. It's a way of learning not to let situations get on top of one but to become a better person because of them. As the meaning of one's existence becomes increasingly clear, so too does the need to trust and to get out of one's own way!

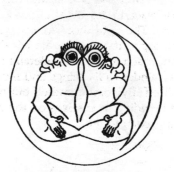

GO WITHIN TO FIND OUT WHAT TO DO.

TIP

Stepping ahead towards one's dreams involves adapting en route and learning from others but never leaning on them.

12 If the shoe fits, think twice about wearing it!

PUTTING THE FOOT IN IT

Shoes represent the boundaries and outlines imposed by family and society, which generally result in the painful need to conform and measure up to some unbelievable expectations. Problems start when forcing oneself to fit into worn-out belief systems that are no longer suitable. Uniform shoes are a classic example of how shoes are used to make everybody think alike and move ahead in an orderly and predetermined manner. It's the dire consequences of doing this that deform feet, for fear of putting a foot wrong. Even though shoes are sorely blamed for foot disorders, they are not the cause; they merely accentuate tense, problematic areas, which, in turn, reflect discomfort that is already in the body. This is why the shoe needs to be on the right foot when it comes to apportioning blame.

Foot disorders are a sign of being way off track with one's soul's purpose. Each pair of shoes reveal the two sides of one's personality, which, if very different, can make putting the shoe on the other foot extremely uncomfortable. Non-conformists and rebels, for instance, are likely to feel out of place in the shoes of a goody-two-shoes, who never puts a foot wrong. The right shoe conveys the marks and impressions of the journey to date, whilst the left shoe reveals whether the current approach to life is accelerating or hampering process. Shoes are a reminder to fix things and mend one's ways, before the bottoms fall off. By sorting oneself out on the outside, things start fixing and mending themselves on the inside, helped along by a changed approach to life.

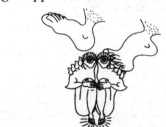

SHOES HIGHLIGHT INNER DISCOMFORT.

WORN OUT SOLES

Feet show how impressed, or otherwise, they are with the choice of shoes. They are quick to complain if footwear is unsuitable or if it hits a sore spot, which then draws attention to a painful memory that still gets in the way. Shoes leave marks on feet showing what's going on beneath the surface. Yet feet are just as capable of leaving their impression on shoes, to the extent that it is often possible to read and interpret footwear in the same way as feet. Footwear take on the nuances of the mind via the feet. Wherever there is a swelling on the foot, there could be a corresponding indentation or worn-out area on the inside of the shoe, with the outer soles of the shoes more likely following the contours of the feet.

- Toes make a mark on shoes when:
  - mentally weighed down
  - heavily concerned
  - wishing to make a deep impression
  - wanting to get one's own ideas across.
- Parts on the shoes can become so worn that they can make a hole, sabotaging progress from the inside out, due to:
  - being worn out and totally exhausted
  - feeling incomplete or that something is missing
  - being weary of protecting oneself by building up extra layers of skin on the feet.
- Footwear falls apart when:
  - coming apart at the seams
  - stretched beyond one's limits
  - needing more space in which to expand.
- The soles of shoes come off due to:
  - doing away with the old to make way for the new
  - needing a different approach to life
  - going through a personal transition
  - needing a new lease of life.
- Scuffed areas on shoes show:
  - where one is scraping through
  - areas of conflict, friction or contention
- Creases highlight areas of concern
- Images and markings speak for themselves (see page 107).

If shoes keep falling apart, it is best to throw them out because they signify the difficulty in keeping life together! Meanwhile the length of time that shoes last is determined by one's attitude. They wear out far more quickly when constantly on the move, whilst they have an even shorter lifespan when dragging the feet or kicking the heels. Meanwhile those dreaded hand-me-downs can be excruciatingly uncomfortable, especially when the previous owner had a very different way of thinking. It really does seem to be insane to wear tight-fitting shoes that scrunch and imprison the toes, whilst keeping a lid on personal ideas. It's little wonder that feet ache at the end of a long, hard day! Kicking off the shoes frees mind, body and soul from self-imposed, social and family restraints and allows one to be oneself.

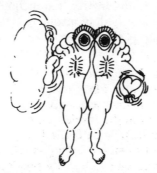

THE BOUNDARIES IMPOSED BY SOCIETY.

FOOT-WEARY ISSUES

Men's footwear is traditionally more practical and sensible and generally provides plenty of support; yet they also keep a great deal of potential well out of sight. Meanwhile women wear anything from the most cumbersome clodhoppers to the daintiest of sandals that are sometimes almost non-existent, as well as the most impractical fashion shoes imaginable that often bear little or no resemblance to the actual shape of their feet. They then have the audacity to complain that their feet hurt!

By putting oneself in one's own shoes it is easy to how see how constrained feet become, especially when they are squeezed into the most outrageous shapes. Yet feet are still expected to act naturally, even though they can barely move a muscle. Fortunately, feet do their best to be accommodating and generally stride out as though nothing out of the ordinary is happening, provided the body is relaxed. Tension immediately restricts and contorts them, bringing problems to the fore, no matter how sensible the shoes are. Shoes use the feet to spell out what the body, mind and soul are complaining about, which is why it is usually such a relief to kick them off, along with all the ridiculous restraints or constrictions that are begrudgingly endured, at the end of a long, hard day. With less pressure on the toes, the mind and body can relax, making it so much easier to think and do things for oneself again.

Meanwhile throwing out shoes is symbolic of letting go of a chapter of one's life, which is why, ideally, all footwear should be dispensed with after a death, divorce, retrenchment and so on, so that a fresh start can be made. Children instinctively know to go barefoot and are intuitively aware of the need to absorb energy from the earth to naturally recharge and revitalize themselves.

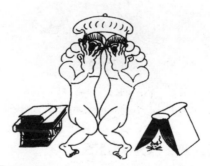

PROBLEMS BROUGHT TO THE FORE BY SHOES.

THE ONWARD JOURNEY

More and more people are turning to nature and natural therapies because they are no longer satisfied with the direction of their lives. They are tired of trying to find answers in the physical world. They yearn for inner peace, yet have forgotten how to be peaceful within themselves. They have had enough of searching for a purpose in life and having no idea of what they are looking for; and they no longer wish to look for the answers to questions that they don't know how to ask. Although there is still a slight reluctance to step out of the comfort zones, along with a fear of what others may think, many are really sick of not being able to be themselves. They no longer wish to hit a brick wall before getting a wake-up call, or to continue to be caught up in artificiality, fickleness and hypocrisy.

Fortunately the massive shift in universal energies is bringing all this, as well as abuse, corruption and deceit, to an end. More and more are turning to the language of the feet to take themselves from the depths of despair and depression, so that they can find their feet and think for themselves again, with the knowledge that the universe is guiding them every step of the way. They soon get to know that the language of the feet is the best gift that they can give themselves and others, since it provides them with the insight needed to reconnect with their authentic self and true spirit. In so doing they have the courage to change, which then inspires others to do the same until, eventually, the world is a better place in which to live. All this and more is only two feet away!

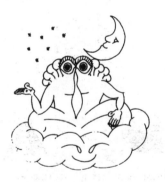

HAPPINESS BEYOND BELIEF!

teach
yourself

reflexology
chris stormer

- Would you like to enjoy the benefits of foot massage?
- Do you want to discover the links between mind and body?
- Are you keen to relieve your tension and improve your health?

Reflexology is an ancient and gentle form of healing that uses reflexes on the feet to increase energy and improve wellbeing, mentally, emotionally and spiritually. Fullly updated and packed with new resources and user-friendly information, **Reflexology** will make sure that you get the most out of this soothing art.

Chris Stormer has worked in the complementary health field for 15 years and is an acknowledged authority on reflexology. She is founder and president of the Academy of Universal Health and Healing and presents workshops worldwide.